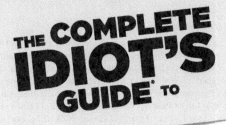

THE COMPLETE IDIOT'S GUIDE® TO

Juice Fasting

D1273149

by Steven Prussack and Bo Rinaldi

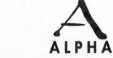

ALPHA

A member of Penguin Group (USA) Inc.

ALPHA BOOKS

Published by Penguin Group (USA) Inc.

Penguin Group (USA) Inc., 375 Hudson Street, New York, New York 10014, USA • Penguin Group (Canada), 90 Eglinton Avenue East, Suite 700, Toronto, Ontario M4P 2Y3, Canada (a division of Pearson Penguin Canada Inc.) • Penguin Books Ltd., 80 Strand, London WC2R 0RL, England • Penguin Ireland, 25 St. Stephen's Green, Dublin 2, Ireland (a division of Penguin Books Ltd.) • Penguin Group (Australia), 250 Camberwell Road, Camberwell, Victoria 3124, Australia (a division of Pearson Australia Group Pty. Ltd.) • Penguin Books India Pvt. Ltd., 11 Community Centre, Panchsheel Park, New Delhi—110 017, India • Penguin Group (NZ), 67 Apollo Drive, Rosedale, North Shore, Auckland 1311, New Zealand (a division of Pearson New Zealand Ltd.) • Penguin Books (South Africa) (Pty.) Ltd., 24 Sturdee Avenue, Rosebank, Johannesburg 2196, South Africa • Penguin Books Ltd., Registered Offices: 80 Strand, London WC2R 0RL, England

Copyright © 2012 by Steven Prussack and Bo Rinaldi

International Standard Book Number: 978-1-61564-225-0
Library of Congress Catalog Card Number: 2012939811

17   16   15   8   7   6   5

Interpretation of the printing code: The rightmost number of the first series of numbers is the year of the book's printing; the rightmost number of the second series of numbers is the number of the book's printing. For example, a printing code of 12-1 shows that the first printing occurred in 2012.

Printed in the United States of America

Note: This publication contains the opinions and ideas of its authors. It is intended to provide helpful and informative material on the subject matter covered. It is sold with the understanding that the authors and publisher are not engaged in rendering professional services in the book. If the reader requires personal assistance or advice, a competent professional should be consulted.

The authors and publisher specifically disclaim any responsibility for any liability, loss, or risk, personal or otherwise, which is incurred as a consequence, directly or indirectly, of the use and application of any of the contents of this book.

Most Alpha books are available at special quantity discounts for bulk purchases for sales promotions, premiums, fund-raising, or educational use. Special books, or book excerpts, can also be created to fit specific needs. For details, write: Special Markets, Alpha Books, 375 Hudson Street, New York, NY 10014.

Publisher: *Mike Sanders*
Executive Managing Editor: *Billy Fields*
Senior Acquisitions Editor: *Brook Farling*
Senior Development Editor: *Christy Wagner*
Senior Production Editor: *Janette Lynn*
Copy Editor: *Jan Zoya*

Cover Designer: *William Thomas*
Book Designers: *William Thomas, Rebecca Batchelor*
Indexer: *Johnna Vanhoose Dinse*
Layout: *Brian Massey*
Senior Proofreader: *Laura Caddell*

Contents

Introduction

This book will empower you to discover how juice fasting can and will transform and improve the quality of your life. Glowing skin, boundless energy, shiny hair, sweet breath, vibrant health, a trim sexy body, and positive disposition are but a few of the side effects you can expect after making juice fasting a part of your lifestyle.

We provide you with a step-by-step program, leaving no stones unturned, guaranteed to be both easy and fun. By following the protocols in this book, you are taking a big step in improving every area of your life. Your body will thank you, as will your mind, spirit, and inner self. We have had incredible results working with clients on restoring their health with juice fasting, and we include awe-inspiring stories of transformation in this book.

The results you'll get from a juice-fasting lifestyle are more effective, long-lasting, and safer than the latest fad diets, going under the knife for expensive surgeries, tummy tucks, and other unnatural and unnecessary treatment modalities.

You may be perplexed on where to begin, what kind of juicer to get, how to make a tasty juice, how to overcome cravings, how to stay motivated, and more. We address all these areas in the following pages. We essentially empower you to become your own doctor, to allow your body to heal itself naturally. We all have healing to do, and there's no better way than with the power and magic of juice fasting.

We get lots of questions about juice fasting. *What if I starve? Can I really live just drinking juices? Can I buy store-bought pasteurized juices for my fast? What if my friends and family think I am crazy?* We cover all this in the following chapters. We wanted to create a book that stands out from all the rest, an updated, down-to-earth prescriptive approach to juice fasting.

You won't find a lot of hype here. We believe the power of juicing speaks for itself. The stories of healing for us and thousands of others also speak for themselves. Are you skeptical? If so, why not give it a chance and see what juice fasting can do for you.

We are confident you are about to turn your world around and create a level of health you never dreamed possible. We want to hear from you! Please email us your stories of transformation. We want to know how this book has helped your life because that was our underlying motivation and intention for writing it.

So sit back, relax, and prepare yourself. We're going to provide everything there is to know about juice fasting, from the history to today. We're thrilled you're about to take this journey with us! May this book answer all your questions and serve as a lifelong guide to your optimum health, growth, beauty, and well-being—all thanks to the power and magic of juice fasting.

Here's to your health! Cheers! Have a juice on us!

How This Book Is Organized

We've written and organized this book to give you the most essential information about juice fasting in a way that's easy to understand.

Chapter 1 gives you the background on juice fasting and why it's so popular today. Chapter 2 provides a step-by-step program for weight loss while Chapter 3 provides the essentials on cleansing and detoxifying your entire body. In Chapters 4 through 6, we offer you a how-to guide on conducting short- and long-term juice fasts along with special tips to target your specific needs. Chapter 7 provides some raw vegan recipes for beginning and ending your fast. And Chapters 8 through 12 provide special juice recipes designed to be incredibly tasty and extremely nutritious. We even included special elixir blends and secret juice recipes, shared for the first time ever!

At the back of the book, we've also included several appendixes full of useful knowledge and information, including a glossary of terms, and extra resources to guide you on your quest for further knowledge of juicing, juice fasting, and nutrition in general. We also include a few stories of transformation from friends all over the planet.

Extras

Throughout the book, we've included little nuggets of extra information. Here's what to look for:

DEFINITION

Turn to these sidebars for definitions of ingredients, juicing terms, and other words you might not be familiar with.

JUICY FACT

In these sidebars, we've included tons of fun facts and bits of additional information.

PULPY PITFALL

For essential tips on things to avoid or beware of when embarking on your juice fast journey, check out these sidebars.

TANTALIZING TIP

These sidebars offer important tips on choosing the right fruit, vegetables, combining ingredients, and more.

Acknowledgments

There are many people to thank, and we are filled with gratitude for the incredible people in our lives.

From Steven: First, I want to thank my co-author Bo Rinaldi for knowing my vision, sharing his knowledge, and being so deeply involved in this project with me. I send deep thanks and gratitude to my agent, Marilyn Allen. Marilyn, you have been incredibly supportive and encouraging, and I know this is the beginning of an incredible working relationship together. Thank you for bringing out the best in me. Deep gratitude to Beryl Greensea, who worked closely with me to bring this book together. Beryl, I truly appreciate your hard work and efforts. Your passion for juice fasting and natural living made this process a true pleasure. I am thrilled we were in alignment to get this message out to the world. To my soul mate and reunited high school sweetheart, my wife, Julie Prussack. You saw my vision right from the beginning and were the only one who believed in me. I am forever filled with gratitude and joy to have you back in my life as my love and best friend. You have joined me on this health journey and discovered the power of juicing for yourself. I am honored to witness your transformation and look forward to a life of love, longevity, and happiness. They say first love never runs dry. Big thanks to my adviser and friend, Dr. Jameth Sheridan. You have been an inspiration and incredibly generous with sharing your vast amount of knowledge and guidance. Thank you for participating in this book and the future we have to spread health and longevity around the world. To you, the reader, I am especially filled with gratitude. Thank you for letting me share this juice-fasting guide with you. May it inspire you and your family to discover the magic and healing of juice fasting. This book would not have been possible without the vision and creative energy of my acquisitions editor, Brook Farling. Thank you so much, Brook, for allowing me to share my passion for juice fasting with the world. You believed in my vision from the start, and I am thrilled to extend my passion into the homes of millions.

From Bo: I want to thank my co-author, Steve Prussack, for his love, passion, and joy for juicing. We are in alignment with bringing our message of transformation and love to the world. This is the first of many projects together, and I look forward to the next. To the love of my life, the brightest light I have ever known, Star Rinaldi. I was blessed the day I met you and I am forever in your grace as your beauty and wisdom feed me the one ingredient we all need the most, love. Big thanks also to Beryl Greensea, who worked closely with us to create the important components of this book.

Trademarks

Juice Fasting Can Change Your Life

In This Chapter

- Why juice fasting works
- The benefits of juice fasting
- The healing qualities of juice fasting
- Juice fasting for everyone? Almost!

Have you ever wondered if you could benefit from a juice fast? Have you considered the possibility that juice fasting could actually *change* your life? Before you answer, first ask yourself these questions:

> *Do I want an efficient way to reach my ideal weight?*
>
> *Do I suffer from any acute or chronic health problems?*
>
> *Do I feel lethargic and older than my years?*
>
> *Am I in touch with what my body needs to thrive?*

If you answered "yes" to one or more of these questions, juice fasting can and will transform and improve the quality of your life.

A juice fast bathes your cells in a flood of nutrition while helping you drop unwanted weight and elevating you to optimal health. It brings you into alignment with the strong, vibrant body you were meant to live in. This powerful rejuvenation method is the ideal way to reset your health on every level.

Juice fasting revamps your digestive, circulatory, lymph, and endocrine systems so they all work in perfect harmony. At the same time, it provides your body with a much-needed break from the laborious process of digesting complex solid foods. It brings vitality and vigor to every part of your body. As your weight gets closer to your personal ideal, you'll discover a new luster to your hair, skin, and nails. Your eyes will become brighter, and your breath will smell fresher—even first thing in the morning! This type of fasting also alleviates depression and fatigue. It makes you feel light and puts a spirited pep in your step as you unleash boundless amounts of energy.

Periodic juice fasting is the most simple and natural way to reach your health goals and shape your body. And you'll find that you begin your transformation fairly rapidly. This is *not* too good to be true. We assure you, it works!

Why Juice Fasting?

Juice fasting has seen an incredible rise in popularity in recent years, even attracting mainstream curiosity and appeal. And with good reason—regular juice fasts are a reliable method for prolonging youthful appearance while keeping lean and fit.

Juice fasting isn't just some new health fad or unfounded natural remedy based on quackery either. In truth, more and more Western doctors are touting the benefits of regular juice fasting as an indispensable part of a safe and effective preventative health-care program. These doctors are recommending juice fasting as an adjunct therapy for the prevention of and treatment for many of the health challenges we face today.

Over the last century, juice fasting has been the preferred method for alleviating and eliminating disease throughout many European countries. Hundreds of health spas throughout Europe offer guided juice fasts as an integral aspect of their healing programs. These spas are a far cry from the fluff-and-buff spas you'll find sprinkled throughout the United States, as their programs are specifically developed for clients seeking natural relief from a wide variety of ailments.

JUICY FACT

The word *spa* refers to a healing center that offers health treatments like hydrotherapy as a curative modality for disease. In Europe, spas focus more on focused healing and reversing disease. It's common to find juice fasting as a core feature of the recommended health protocols in these spas. In the United States, however, we find that the term *spa* is used to describe a facility that offers luxury services such as massages, facials, and other superficial treatments that promote temporary well-being, but not necessarily healing on a deep level.

Juice fasting is finally receiving mainstream appeal and serious recognition in the United States. Since its introduction in the late 1800s by several health pioneers, juice fasting has caught on and experienced a surge in growth over the past several decades. The floodgates to juice-fasting know-how have been opened and what once was a trickle is now becoming an unstoppable force of self-healing and personal empowerment!

Many new books, movies, internet resources, infomercials, and word-of-mouth information document the power and magic of juice fasting and its innumerable benefits. Juice fasting will only continue to gain credence from the medical community as more and more people become living proof of the transformation it makes to your health and appearance.

Possibly the best news of all is that *you* can juice fast. Yes, you! Nearly anyone can enjoy the amazing rejuvenation a juice fast brings. In fact, it's so safe and easy to do, all you need is the information in this book and the desire to look and feel your best.

If you're relatively healthy, you don't have to hesitate before starting your first juice-fasting program after reading through the important information in this book. However, if you take prescription medications or have a significant health issue, we recommend visiting your medical practitioner for a check-up and discussing your desire to juice fast before starting one of our programs. Your doctor should be able to wean you off your medications as you become healthy and in balance again.

Juice Fasting Works!

Fasting is the most universal, logical, and instinctual method of healing found in the natural world. It permeates the entire animal kingdom. In fact, fasting is something our animal counterparts do with great regularity. Bears hibernate for months without eating, living entirely off their fat stores. Lions often eat only once a week. And large snakes can live an entire year between meals.

If you're a parent, you probably know how common it is for a toddler or young child to simply refuse food for several days at a time and for reasons that may be mysterious to you. But you might be surprised to find that if you offer him a fresh pressed organic juice during his boycott on food, he'll drink it. It's futile to push solid food on a fasting child because the protest will just become an unpleasant battle of wills, but offering fresh juice is a brilliant way to ensure he speeds his healing while still getting some essential nutrition during his self-imposed fast.

Many children instinctively know when their bodies need to eat and when they need to rest. You possess the same inborn capacity, but to recover and hone this skill, you'll need to cleanse your body enough to restore the intuition necessary for decoding the subtle—and not-so-subtle—messages your body sends you. The vast majority of us are completely out of touch with the signals our bodies send us because of the accumulated pollutants we harbor and our ability to pay attention to our gut feelings and instincts has long been impaired.

JUICY FACT

Your nervous system doesn't just send messages from your brain to your body. You also have a network of neural tissue—called the enteric nervous system—centralized in the abdominal region that sends messages to your brain and the rest of your body. This second or "gut brain" has its own senses and is responsible for those butterflies in your stomach and your gut reactions.

It would do us all well to get out of the mindless habit of eating three square meals a day riddled with heavy foods. We'd all be in better health if we practiced eating lightly sometimes and juice fasting regularly rather than gorging every time our tummies grumble or the clock tells us it's mealtime. Lightening our digestive burden really does wonders for alleviating all kinds of health problems, and juice fasting can be a wonderful way to recover from many common complaints.

Every time you juice fast, you'll notice a great improvement in your overall health and well-being. Even just a 1-day fast can do wonders. If you start making healthy diet changes and commit to juice fasting regularly, you'll give your health a total overhaul in a short period of time.

Juice fasting works so well for healing illness and supporting wellness because it releases your body from the burden of constant digestion and gives your organs the chance to flush out all those accumulated toxins. Developing a regular habit of taking a break from eating solid food offers your tired, overworked body some very needed and deserved rest. When you add fresh organic juices to this scenario, you have a recipe for vast improvement in your health!

Taking Your Health in Your Own Hands

Each of us is born with a body that constantly strives to maintain balance and *homeostasis*. Use this fact to your advantage, and take your health and healing into your own hands! The innate healing power your body holds has been unjustly minimized by Western medicine and its theories on disease. But disease is just that, *dis-ease*. It's a state that reflects imbalance. It's not that there's something inherently wrong or permanently flawed in your body; it's that there's something obstructing your natural state of health.

The symptoms of most diseases are an expression of your body doing what it was designed to do: destroying an obstruction and bringing balance to your body. A fever is designed to kill viruses and bacteria, a cough is produced to remove an irritant, and even tumors are the result of the body pressing accumulated toxins into a single mass so they don't overload and destroy your vital organs.

Your body is an amazingly intelligent entity all on its own. Imagine the changes when your body starts receiving its own crucial messages and follows the plan accordingly. The point when you consciously choose to foster a healthy relationship with your body through juice fasting, is when you'll unleash the power of your *enteric nervous system* and experience a level of intuition you never knew possible! Juice fasting relieves this neural tissue, located in your abdomen, of its usual occupation engrossed in constantly regulating the flow of gastric juices and releasing nutrients into your blood stream while moving food through your digestive system. This frees your enteric nervous system to be more useful for the other important activities it coordinates in your body.

DEFINITION

Homeostasis, which translates to "standing still," refers to your body's ability to heal itself in order to maintain equilibrium. Your **enteric nervous system** is your second brain. This "gut brain" is normally busy directing digestive duties, but it also helps you react to sudden stimulus. When you jump from a jolting surprise or retract your hand from a hot object, your enteric nervous system is involved in these instinctual processes. It also moderates your mood and can be stimulated to relieve depression.

Your "gut brain" gives you that funny feeling when you know something isn't right but can't find a logical explanation for it. It also largely regulates your state of mind. Nearly all the nerve fibers in the vagus nerve—responsible for the communication between your organs and your brain—send messages from your gut to your brain rather than the other way around. What's amazing is that the vagus nerve can be stimulated to alleviate depression, which further reinforces the fact that depression arises from imbalances in your digestive system.

When you eat a heavy meal, you may feel an initial sense of satisfaction, but it ends up creating pressure on your internal organs and exhausts your digestive system. In turn, you produce less of those happy chemicals like serotonin and get caught in a negative cycle where overeating brings an initial state of relief but eventually leaves you feeling somewhat depressed or stoic. Rather than letting these organs do their full round of duties, they get caught in a loop of digestive and cleansing processes and can't devote their usefulness to their other important tasks.

All this attests to the vital connection between what you eat and how you feel. When you eat foods that are hard to digest, you waste precious energy and sabotage your body's effort to self-regulate. On the other hand, when you eat simple foods—and better yet, when you juice fast—you foster communication between your body and brain and actually increase your capacity for happiness! This is part of the reason many people find they feel incredible and have tons of energy while juice fasting.

Be proactive about your health. Use juice fasting as a tool for managing your ongoing self-improvement and healing journey. Let the protocols we offer in this book guide you toward your own state of optimal health. It's very empowering to realize that *you* are responsible for achieving perfect health and harmony. Use this realization to your fullest benefit.

Juice Fast Benefits

So let's get more specific here. What exactly are the benefits of juice fasting? It's entirely conceivable that they're so numerous that listing each one would encompass an entire book. To give you a basic understanding, though, we can tell you that it will certainly bring you health and vibrancy in ways you've never known.

To begin with, you'll experience a surge in your energy levels. You'll start to lose excess weight, or you may even gain a bit if you're already underweight. Your skin will take on a luminous, clear, and glowing complexion, while your nails become smooth and sturdy. Even your hair can regain its color—reversing the graying process—and will grow thicker and shinier with less breakage. You can also expect dramatic improvements in acute or chronic illnesses of all kinds. Our juice fasts have cured us of such varied illnesses and problems like migraine headaches, mood swings, metabolic issues, and the numerous symptoms associated with poor digestion. This is a big part of the reason we're so passionate about juice fasting!

After a juice fast, you'll look and feel lighter, like you just came from a relaxing vacation. Friends, colleagues, and family members will start asking you what your secret is to turning back the clock. Even just one short 3- or 7-day juice fast can make you feel and look dramatically different.

TANTALIZING TIP

Here's a fun little tidbit you can include in your daily beauty regimen. (Men, you can give it a try, too!) Many fruits and vegetables contain properties that exfoliate the skin, tighten pores, and help heal acne. Give yourself a home spa treatment by mixing a bit of pineapple juice or wheatgrass into a clay mask, or use your juice pulp as an additive to an oatmeal mask. Take advantage of those natural enzymes and potent skin rejuvenators.

But you don't have to go on a vacation to find yourself so rejuvenated! Even if you're going about your normal life while juice fasting, your body is taking some time off. Surprisingly, that little time can do wonders for melting away years of accumulated stress.

The lasting power of these amazing health improvements varies, depending on a few factors. The length of your fast, how often you fast, the way you begin and end your fast, and your overall lifestyle choices between fasting all factor into the end results you'll see and feel. You have to decide whether you want your juice fast to give your health a temporary upgrade or offer a new standard to live by.

As with most things, you get out of juice fasting what you put into it. Here lies the key to superb health and well-being, and it's yours for the taking. Many people have completely healed themselves from minor ills and even the most serious diseases by juice fasting. It's so powerful, in fact, that if you juice fast regularly, you can eventually wean yourself off of pharmaceutical drugs. We recommend consulting with your physician before making that decision, but juice fasting will balance your body while restoring health.

Juice fasting often succeeds where other therapies have failed. It can knock out persistent antibiotic-resistant infections, stop a cold in its tracks, and put an end to constant recurring headaches. Juice fasting has proven to be effective in safely healing many chronic diseases such as lupus, arthritis, and asthma.

Take comfort that after several fasts you'll finally attain your ideal weight. You'll be toning your insides and toning your outer appearance as well. Pounds will begin to melt away, and in their place, you'll find the extra energy you've been missing. A strong commitment to lifestyle improvements and the support of juice fasting will make this weight change a permanent one rather than a roller coaster of gain and loss. Weight-loss management with juice fasting releases unwanted pounds the *right* way, by encouraging your body to heal itself and rely on rich nutritional sources for energy rather than store fat.

PULPY PITFALL

Many diseases and metabolic disorders such as diabetes can make juice fasting a tricky endeavor. If you have a preexisting condition for which you're currently receiving medical attention, please consult with your primary care provider before embarking on a juice fast.

If you're concerned about your willpower and committing to a juice fast, take heart that our first juice fasts only lasted anywhere from 1 to 3 days. Now our fasts might last 20 days or more, and it's become so easy and enjoyable that the hardest part is stopping! In fact, this entire book was written while we were both doing extended juice fasts because we find it helps clear our minds and leads to maximum productivity.

There's nothing wrong with taking it slowly as you introduce yourself to the world of juice fasting. Doing so can give you the confidence you need to succeed in your efforts, time and time again. If you feel like you're out of balance, suffering uncomfortable symptoms, and aren't sure how to find relief, try a juice fast. If you feel like you have low energy and want to feel more vibrant *now*, try a juice fast. And if you're searching for inspiration for a major overhaul of your life and want to eliminate old habits, try a juice fast.

It's time to propel yourself into an intuitive, quick-thinking, flexible, fast-moving new you. Yes, you can be a superhero! Are you ready for the change?

Safe, Fast, and Effective

Juice fasting is safe, fast, and very effective. It draws out the healing principles inherent to your body and uses them to their fullest potential. This is the reason why even after your first juice cleanse, you should notice immediate differences in your health.

This isn't some extreme or dangerous diet. It has no side effects—unless you consider great health a side effect! It's simply a way to give your body a break so it can do some major damage control.

Juice fasting is the most nutrient-rich, calorie-restricted diet one can go on, minus all the bulk that consumes energy for digestion. If you're familiar with diet programs, you probably know that most of them are variations of calorie-restriction diets. The idea is that eating fewer calories than your body needs for its daily energy requirements burns fat and helps you lose weight. This is certainly true of juice fasting, but you have some added elements that are essential to this process.

Calorie restriction isn't just useful for weight loss; it's also an essential component of healing in general. Because fresh-pressed juices are fundamentally concentrated liquid nutrition, they meet your body's needs for vitamins, minerals, and other phytonutrients and keep your body's pH balanced. The potent phytochemicals in your fresh juices are immediately ready to go to work healing your tissues and assisting proper cell functioning and they're packed with enzymes that collaborate with your cells in healing and maintaining your health and metabolism on a cellular level.

Perhaps you've heard of the benefits of maintaining an alkaline pH-balanced body? Fresh juices are incredibly high in the essential and trace minerals that perfectly balance your electrolytes and keep your blood pH slightly alkaline. The human body thrives optimally with a blood pH between 7.2 and 7.8. When you juice fast, your body naturally becomes alkaline as a result of the high mineral content in fresh juices. An alkaline system oxygenates your blood, providing better *cellular respiration.*

DEFINITION

Cellular respiration refers to the metabolic processes within a cell. This includes the conversion of nutrients into energy, which fuels other cellular activity, and the removal of waste products.

When your body is alkaline, you stop craving addictive substances like coffee, tobacco, and chocolate. In fact, the physical addiction to such substances is a cry from your body for alkaline minerals!

But juice fasting is the only natural, safe, and incredibly effective way to replace your old crutches—like caffeine—with real energy-supporting nutrients while aiding and maintaining harmony in your body. It's the only way to drop serious amounts of weight quickly without damaging your organs. And it's the perfect nutrition therapy for balancing deficiencies.

Bringing Out Your Inner Beauty

Who doesn't want to look young, healthy, vibrant, and sexy? It's natural for us to be attracted to people with these qualities, and we all have the desire to embody them. What could possibly be sexier than a healthy, clean, lean, and fully functioning human body? When you purify your inside, you beautify your outside!

When your body has the opportunity to remove the burden of accumulated toxins, your energy dramatically increases. This store of vital energy surging through your freshly enlivened and renewed body will instantly make you more attractive. When you feel good, you look good, and people respond positively to those with tons of vibrant energy.

The healing *phytochemicals* in your enzyme-rich juices will tone your skin and give it a supple, rich luster. Fine lines will gradually fade away, and your skin will emanate a golden glow all its own. Acne, eczema, and psoriasis may begin to improve almost overnight and can be eliminated completely through regular periodic fasting.

DEFINITION

Phytochemicals are the colored and sometimes colorless pigments in your fruits and vegetables. They're responsible for protecting plants from predators and the elements as well as healing tissue damage. They often act as antioxidants, and impart all these benefits to their consumers.

Because of the obvious calorie restriction, you can naturally assume you'll see impressive weight loss during a single juice fast or through a series of these cleanses. Juice fasting is not a miracle fix-it system for removing every bit of excess fat overnight. But it can offer concentrated periods of time to melt away the fat through a series of short juice fasts. Accompanying your fasts with an overall change in your eating habits is the best way to make these changes permanent.

Countless testimonials indicate juice fasting can restore color to graying hair and reverse balding by stimulating brand-new hair growth. The chlorophyll in green juices and wheatgrass juice are particularly noted as being potent remedies for graying and thinning hair, but other helpful juices include carrot and Indian gooseberry.

A healthy body is a sexual body. It's obvious to assume that when in perfect health, *all* our faculties for pleasure should be in perfect working order. Juice fasting cleanses, lubricates, and tones the glandular system, making it the ultimate natural approach to sexual rejuvenation. When you remove the impurities that clog your arteries and slow down blood flow, you restore balance to your circulatory system. This alone leads to the rediscovery of your natural vigor and healthy libido.

Feeling sexy *is* sexy, and having confidence in your optimally functioning body is supremely attractive.

Total Regeneration

Juice fasting doesn't need to be restricted to those wishing to cure an existing ailment. It really is the best type of preventative care available for staving off illness during any stage of life.

Juice fasting is incredible for maintaining good health through the cold and flu season. It both supports and helps rebuild the immune system so well you'll no longer need to line up at the pharmacy for a seasonal flu vaccine. When you begin to feel a slight tickle in your throat or notice you're making unhealthy food choices, it's a great idea to embark on a short-term juice fast to bring yourself back into alignment with perfect health.

All health challenges, including diseases of the mind and body, are due to imbalances. These imbalances can be the result of nutritional deficiencies or an excess of certain nutrients. They can be caused by pollutants in your food and environment or they can be the result of a sluggish digestive system that isn't able to fully do its job.

The point is that our bodies aren't designed to be sick, and our cells aren't designed to die before completing their various life cycles. Toxins stored in our cells and introduced via our food, air, and water interfere with normal cell functioning and cause corruption and cell death. This, in turn, leads to all types of diseases and premature aging. An acidic pH, overgrowth of fungal forms like *Candida albicans*, plus toxins stored in your tissues all push the "composting" button in your body to the limit. They start breaking down your body and prematurely decomposing it! These are the factors that lead to degenerative diseases and premature aging and death.

JUICY FACT

Your intestinal lining only takes between two days and one month to completely regenerate, as does your skin. Your red blood cells are completely new after four months. Even your muscles and bones are completely cellularly regenerated every three and four years, respectively.

Drinking fresh juices as the backbone for a cleansing fast promotes a life-enhancing state of alkalinity and supports longevity. It halts the "composting" process and cleans out your cells. It helps regenerate damage done to organs like your liver and pancreas and can help regenerate the lining of your stomach. There are even reports of people healing cavities and growing new enamel on their teeth after prolonged or frequent juice fasting. It shouldn't come as a surprise that a majority of the cells in our bodies are regenerated every 7 to 10 years. That means in just a few years, you almost have a completely different body! That's the power and intelligence of the human body.

Your cells *want* to regenerate—it's their sole purpose in existence. And your body *wants* to remain in balance. Disease is not a natural state of being, and it's not inevitable, either. It's simply the result of inadequate living conditions. Juice fasting is the solution for regenerating your good health.

The Fountain of Youth

Your body came with a blueprint that will keep it in perfect working order for upward of 200 years. Most of us never experience our real potential because we've become weakened from the effects of stress, toxins in our diet, and pollution in the environment. Health is the natural state of being for all living things. Our modern lifestyle has damaged our quality of life. And this has led to premature aging, decreasing our natural joy and thirst for life. This is all easily remedied once we're empowered with the right tools, which begins with the practice of juice fasting.

The environmental toxins we've been talking about are also known as *free radicals*, and they essentially eat away the health of your cells. Free radicals attach themselves to your cell membranes, and after time, they weaken and destroy your cell walls, causing accelerated aging due to tissue breakdown. They're also one of the main factors of disease.

Thankfully, juicing and juice fasting provide a solution. Fresh fruit and vegetable juices are loaded with enzymes and antioxidants that neutralize harmful free radicals and reverse their damaging effects. Once restored, your cells are free to continue their regular maintenance jobs without being attacked or hindered by free radicals. Through regular juice fasting, it's entirely possible to slow down and even reverse the aging process for a very significant amount of time. This alone should tell you how invaluable juicing is for your body.

TANTALIZING TIP

Remember that fresh juices in any combination are a healthy addition to your diet as a whole. Incorporate them into your daily meal plan to boost your daily nutrition. You can also prepare your mind for juice fasting by replacing one of your meals during the day with a large, 32-ounce juice.

Who would have thought that the modern-day juicer would prove to be the eternally sought-after fountain of youth? As it turns out, the hidden components of vibrantly colored plants offer us the key to natural longevity and good health. Nature has provided all we need to maintain optimal health, so why go under the knife or take pills to try to make yourself look younger? You can do it all yourself, naturally, with juice fasting! Fresh fruit and vegetable juices supply your body with the essential vitamins, minerals, and nutrients it needs to truly thrive!

Juice Fasting Through the Ages

Anecdotal evidence exists that juice fasting was an important aspect of ancient Indian *Ayurvedic* treatments as far back as 5,000 years ago. In particular, Panchakarma—a cleansing and rejuvenating program for the body, mind, and consciousness—included daily massage, purging treatments, and fasting with the aid of various herbal concoctions incorporated into a base of fruit juice. Such ancient juice protocols included mango juice, Indian gooseberry, and other fruits that were prescribed depending on a person's body type and specific malady.

DEFINITION

Ayurveda is an ancient Indian healing art that translates as the "science of longevity." It has been relied upon for approximately 5,000 years as a system that restores health based on bringing an individual into harmony with nature. It provides guidance regarding food and lifestyle so healthy people stay healthy and people with health challenges can improve their health.

In ancient times, fasting was recognized as the safest and most efficient way to heal the sick. Despite the introduction of pills and surgical procedures as the "go-to" cures in our culture, fasting remains the best way to maintain, preserve, or restore health.

Countless religious and other historical figures and modern medical professionals have extolled the many benefits of fasting, including the ancient philosophers Pythagoras and Plato, who fasted for greater mental and physical efficiency. Some of the most prominent religious figures such as Jesus Christ, Moses, Mohammad, and the Buddha promoted the benefits of fasting for both spiritual and bodily purification.

Modern Medical Integration

Juice fasting really began its solid transformation of the health movement in the early 1900s. It has its roots set deeply in the development of naturopathic medicine, although most practitioners of the time were in fact medical doctors. The father of naturopathic medicine, Dr. Arnold Ehret (1866–1922), is quoted as saying "Fasting is the master key to mental and spiritual unfoldment and evolution." This might seem like a lofty claim, but it's truly an accurate one.

Ehret isn't alone in his assertions. Thanks to the many doctors—like Dr. Otto Buchinger, Dr. Norman Walker, Dr. Max Gerson, and countless others—who were committed to integrity and finding real solutions to difficult health challenges, we're now able to take juice fasting into the mainstream. Their intuition and hard work laid the path for a medical revelation whose time has come!

PULPY PITFALL

It's important to distinguish the differences between water fasting and juice fasting. Water fasting was the most common method of fasting for centuries and is still used during religious practices. The difference is prolonged water fasting requires total rest and strict supervision by a medical practitioner to be sure it's done safely. For this reason, we recommend juice fasting as the superior method to support self-empowered detox and complete body rejuvenation.

In today's medical community, juice fasting isn't just some archaic alternative therapy but one that has the promise of revolutionizing our entire approach to health and healing. The results are in, and they're overwhelmingly positive. This is something the medical community cannot ignore, and we're now on the verge of changing the ways doctors treat disease.

We continue to find countless physicians who know and support the benefits of juice fasting. For example, Dr. Joel Fuhrman has written numerous books on the benefits of juice fasting to lose weight and reverse disease. He even prescribes vegetable juice fasting as part of his anticancer solution protocol. He even goes as far as to say that "The time may come when not offering this substantially more effective nutritional approach (juice fasting) will be considered mal-practice." This is possibly the most poignant statement ever made by a doctor on the subject of juice fasting!

Rudolph Ballentine, MD; Elson Haas, MD; Allan Cott, MD; Gabriel Cousens, MD; and Dr. Richard Schultz all extoll the immense health and healing benefits of juice fasting and use it in practical applications with their own clients with great success. They've each aided individuals to heal from nearly every malady, from cancer to diabetes, and heart disease to psoriasis.

TANTALIZING TIP

Find a doctor who will be supportive of your efforts to juice fast. Chances are that if your doctor doesn't agree with juice fasting as a method of healing, he or she just hasn't been well educated about its incredible healing potential. Your doctor can't recommend something unfamiliar, so search around and be sure to find a practitioner who is supportive.

Many medical and naturopathic doctors use juice fasting to treat symptoms and reverse a multitude of diseases with great success. Is your doctor open to the idea of recommending juice fasting and other natural remedies as opposed to prescription medication? If not, perhaps it's time to seek the advice of a practitioner with an understanding of natural healing systems.

Who Can Juice Fast?

So who can do a juice fast? Nearly anyone! Of course, there are a few exceptions to this rule. In general, children shouldn't juice fast unless they're simply refusing to eat on their own and you're encouraging them to drink fresh juices. Growing children need calories and adequate sustenance to support their expanding bodies and should never be forced to juice fast.

Juice fasting really isn't a great idea for pregnant or breast-feeding mothers. It's far more supportive to add fresh juices to your diet when in these phases of life. Pregnant and nursing mothers need calories to support the nutritional demands of the child relying on them for sustenance. Plus, the detoxification a juice fast brings can pass those toxins to your child. When you remove these substances from your tissues, they enter your blood and lymph system to be released. As they circulate in the blood stream, they pass on to your baby in utero or via your breast milk.

If you hope to become pregnant in the future, however, juice fasting is an ideal choice for lightening your toxic load and preventing these poisons from being passed on to your child. (We cover this topic more in Chapter 3.)

TANTALIZING TIP

Children should not be encouraged to take a long break from eating solids—unless there's some medical reason for this—but they sometimes refuse to eat on their own free will. Encourage your child to drink fresh juices during these times to ensure they're still getting the nutrition they need.

For those on kidney dialysis or with diabetes and other such illnesses, juice fasting may indeed help manage your symptoms or even reverse your condition, but doing so may be difficult to navigate. We never recommend the immediate cessation of your current therapies or medications unless approved by your health-care professional. We also recommend you enlist the help of a supportive doctor if you want to use juice fasting as a method for curing your condition.

Otherwise, anyone can enjoy the multitude of benefits juice fasting offers. You can do it! You can reverse your chronic illness. You can help speed recovery from an injury. Start a juice-fasting regimen to reach your long-term weight-loss goals. Clear your skin of acne and tone your skin to remove wrinkles by juice fasting. Extend your life and make it enjoyable. Juice fast regularly so you always look and feel your best for all your long life!

The Least You Need to Know

- You can take control of your own health with juice fasting.
- Juice fasting is a safe, fast, and effective method for improving your health.
- Your body can regenerate damaged cells and organs during a juice fast.
- Juice fasting alleviates depression.
- You can increase your longevity by juice fasting regularly.
- Juice fasting is an ancient method of healing many modern doctors support.
- Nearly anyone can safely perform a juice fast.

Juice Fasting for Weight Loss

Chapter 2

In This Chapter

- Juice fasting for weight loss
- Long-term weight management
- Feeding your body on a cellular level
- Cleansing fast programs

One of the most popular reasons to embark on a fast, of any kind, is weight loss. We may intuitively abstain from food due to a lack of hunger or try to eat light for a few days to try getting a handle on weight gain. Others may go on a specialized diet plan where they track and restrict the number of calories they consume each day while eating packaged diet meals and snacks that come along with their chosen program. These types of calorie restrictions may be commonly used for releasing excess weight, but juice fasting gives this process a well-needed and much improved makeover.

The problem with going on a diet and replacing normal food with diet snacks is that these calorie-restricted diet foods are devoid of any real nutrition. Although some might temporarily fill your belly, they don't nourish your body in any substantial way. Instead, these low-calorie foodstuffs are nothing more than cellulose and toxic chemicals with artificial flavoring. If you've ever tried such foods, you know you're usually still hungry after eating them.

There's nothing wrong with limiting your calories to lose a few pounds, as long as you're providing your body the nutrition it requires. With a juice fast, you do just that.

Juice Fast to Lose Weight Fast

When it comes to healthy weight loss, there's no miracle pill or diet. However, juice fasting is the perfect way to obtain consistent and dramatic results for permanent long-term weight loss.

JUICY FACT

Poor food choices are only one cause of common nutrient deficiencies. In addition, our soils have been depleted by farming methods like mono cropping and pesticide use. This practice continues to kill essential living organisms in the soil and makes minerals unavailable for plants to absorb. Juicing is a perfect way to up your nutrient intake. It's essential that you use only organically grown fruits and vegetables during your juice cleanse.

How much weight you'll lose depends on the length of your fast and, just as importantly, the lifestyle choices you make following your fast. If you start off with a 1-week juice fast, you can expect to shed a few pounds. On the other hand, a shorter 3-day fast will help you lose an average of up to three pounds. You could certainly experience dramatic results from a long-term month-long juice fast, but you don't have to go to this extreme to shed excess pounds. Ultimately, fasting regularly and intermittently throughout the months and years as part of an ongoing healthy lifestyle will deliver the most powerful, permanent results.

Remember, juice fasting isn't just the latest diet fad. It's the best way to improve your health and discover the beautiful body you already have, and in this book, we set you up to make a complete positive lifestyle change. By choosing to juice fast, you're making a serious commitment to your health. We encourage you to use this period of dramatic weight loss to catapult into a lifestyle that supports your naturally slim and energetic new body.

Reaching Your Weight-Loss Goals Naturally

It's important that you have the right mind-set about juice fasting before you begin. We want you to have full confidence that this is not a starvation diet. Juice fasting provides your body with incredible nutrition while *restricting* your caloric intake.

You most assuredly will be consuming some calories during your fast, although it will be less than what you're used to. You'll have enough *macronutrients* to give you plenty of energy and support your body in carrying out its normal metabolic processes. This is a time of cleansing and releasing, so you won't be actively building new muscle or storing fat. The amount of juice we recommend drinking throughout the day ensures that you're always well fed and never hungry. In fact, we could call this a juice *feast*, rather than a fast! You will always be nourished on our programs.

DEFINITION

Macronutrients are nutrients that provide caloric value. Carbohydrates, protein, and fat are macronutrients as opposed to *micronutrients,* which provide vitamins, minerals, and enzymes.

When you're juice fasting, your body will function more efficiently. You begin improving the function of your body on a cellular level, which encourages deep removal of the accumulated toxins embedded in your body's fatty tissue. Many of the recommended juices in this book were carefully chosen to optimally assist your body in efficiently cleansing the colon and removing the stagnant waste that slows down your elimination.

You may notice that your weight loss seems dramatic at the beginning of your juice fast but then may plateau. The fat loss at the beginning is more accelerated because you are eliminating stored waste early on in your fast, and any subsequent weight loss after this initial stage is actual fat melting away. During a longer fast, you can expect to lose an average of about 1 pound per day. Losing weight at this rate is quite rapid weight loss, so please don't try to push yourself to lose more than this by altering your juice-fasting program. Just stick with it, and you'll see amazing results in just a short time.

Regular Maintenance Is Key

The key to long-term weight maintenance is to juice fast regularly while consistently maintaining proper eating habits. It's great to practice juice fasting one day a week or three days a month. How often you fast depends on you, your preference, and your lifestyle goals. Keep in mind that if your goal is long-term weight loss, you should commit to continuous conscious care for your health. We recommend working toward a healthy, plant-based diet.

It's unrealistic to assume that a simple 1-day juice fast will help shed more than a few ounces of actual body fat. However, following our important guidelines for beginning your juice fast will spark increased weight loss. We recommend completing several fasts over a period of time as the ideal way to find your perfect weight.

We also recommend challenging yourself with a longer fast when you feel the time is right to obtain a more significant body makeover. This could be a 7-, 14-, or even 28-day juice fast, just do what you feel is right. Longer fasts like these lead to deeper cleansing of your entire body and encourage weight loss. You'll be thrilled to see your body transform so significantly, but it's imperative that you maintain healthy food choices along with your periodic juice fasts to ensure that your results are permanent. If you're trying to lose a large amount of weight, the most effective way to meet your goals is to juice fast intermittently and regularly.

TANTALIZING TIP

Don't worry about weight loss at first. In fact, don't even step on the scale. Chances are you may lose a few pounds during a fast, but they will return if you go straight back to your old eating habits. Instead, focus on the light feeling you get from a juice fast and enjoy the extra energy. Trust that each time you juice fast you are cleaning your insides and helping your body find its ideal weight. Try to improve your overall eating habits after each short juice fast, and you'll have a recipe for long-term success!

Not only does periodic fasting offer your body a series of consistent breaks from solid food and digestive duties, it also helps you develop better eating habits as a whole. As you weave juice fast into your weight loss or health maintenance program, you'll naturally be more attracted to fresh, vibrant food, so shifting your dietary patterns toward healthier choices will become very easy. The reason for this is simple: when you give your body a break during a fast, your being becomes more enlightened, and your body intuitively tells you exactly what it needs. Your tongue becomes cleaner and able to easily decipher and enjoy the natural flavors in food. Soon enough your body will crave only incredibly nutritious foods.

You'll Never Go Hungry!

The irony about juice fasting is that even though you technically won't be *eating* anything, you'll be consuming more concentrated nutrition than your body has ever experienced. It's simply impossible to starve when your nutritional requirements are finally being met or even exceeded.

And then there's the sheer volume of juice you'll be consuming. We recommend you drink four 32-ounce servings of juice throughout the day to keep you nourished, energized, and feeling your best. That measures out to 16 cups of liquid for the day. Any time you feel a hunger pang, just take a sip of some juice and your hunger will subside.

What's more, you'll also begin to distinguish between true hunger and your unhealthy habits of eating for comfort and emotional security, and you'll naturally eliminate food addictions.

The Truth About Hunger

It's likely you'll feel moments of intense hunger during your juice fast. Stick with it, and know that these feelings are mostly psychological and will pass quickly. Understand that fasting isn't the same as starvation. Your intelligent body has specific mechanisms in place to feed itself during times when food is scarce. Your body has a hierarchy of tissues in place it breaks down for energy when in fasting mode. Fortunately, the first tissue your body breaks down and converts to energy is fat. Your body knows accumulated fat isn't necessary or healthy for survival. It wants to get rid of it, when given the chance.

In modern society, we are out of touch with the call of true hunger. The sensations we most often associate with hunger are not actually a signal from the body as a need for food. The stomach growls that sound off as your stomach empties itself and begins to shrink in size are simply that—your stomach emptying and shrinking. Even a feeling of lightheadedness can be due to metabolic imbalances rather than actual hunger. Many of your urges to eat are actually a misunderstood cry for *hydration*. It's highly unlikely that the majority of us are familiar with the actual sensations of hunger. When you get a hunger sensation during your juice fast, drink more juice. A big glass of water works well, too.

JUICY FACT

You don't need to eat three square meals or even six small meals every day to stay healthy. You just need to consume enough calories to keep yourself energized. If you overeat and consume too many calories one day, try a juice fast the next to balance yourself out.

True hunger is completely different from the false hunger pangs you experience when you feel it's time for a meal. When you learn the difference, you'll find your body communicates true hunger in a different way. Don't expect a stomach growl to signal you're really hungry. Say good-bye to the idea of feeling hungry just because the clock says it's lunchtime. Prepare to experience something brand new, more like a full-body sensation that communicates it's time to fuel up.

Because you'll be free from the habits of comfort eating, you'll be able to make better choices about the meals you use to fuel your body. Soon you'll naturally reverse your food addictions and easily make choices that give you satisfaction via nutrition.

During your juice fast, you can expect to experience some cravings. This happens when your body begins to cleanse and release old toxins into the bloodstream. When this happens, the leftover debris from those chips you ate last month or pizza you had last week cause cravings. The remedy is to drink some juice or water and wait it out until they subside. Even though this can be uncomfortable, you should never experience *real* hunger while juice fasting. And take it from us, these cravings subside quickly, sometimes in minutes.

Juicing Is a Feast for Your Cells

Your cells are crying out for real nutrition! Not only that, they're also having difficulty breathing and fueling you with energy because accumulated fats and complex proteins impact their efficiency. Your bloodstream is being slowed because of excess fat in your system. This is a major problem because your blood needs to deliver nutrients throughout your body. Wonder why you often have low energy? Certain fats interact with the same receptor sites carbohydrates use for energy, preventing your cells from being efficient. They get plugged up and aren't able to carry out the metabolic processes necessary for energy production and waste removal.

Drinking fresh vegetable and fruit juice delivers nutrients to every cell in your body quickly and efficiently. Because your body doesn't have to exert much effort to extract the nutrients from juice, you immediately absorb an incredible amount of nutrition. Thanks to juice fasting, heavy fats in your bloodstream will no longer slow down your metabolism. Energy production will flow effortlessly to nourish all your waiting, hungry cells.

TANTALIZING TIP

Your cells make up every muscle, bone, organ, and hair in your body. If you're not feeding your cells, you're not feeding your body. Remember this next time you crave processed foods, and reach for a fresh juice instead!

Cleansing Weight Loss

There's more to losing weight than just dropping a few inches from your waist size. While your body melts away stored fat, it converts it into energy. As you lose weight, you also remove the first layer of defense your body uses to buffer toxins that would overload your organs if allowed to circulate freely. Juice fasting restricts your caloric intake enough to begin burning away those fatty tissues along with the toxins stored deep within.

If you're losing weight, you're also removing toxins from your body. The weight loss is motivating, but what's most exciting is that you're actually getting healthier on the deepest level possible. Removing fat deposits means cleaner blood, healthier organs, and an overall more efficient body system. It means your cells will no longer be overburdened by fats endlessly circulating in your bloodstream, suppressing your energy. Keeping a normal weight is about more than just looking good; it's about feeling extraordinary and being rewarded with optimal health.

The 1-Day Perfect Weight-Loss Prescription

This program was designed as a once-a-week juice fast that safely and quickly helps you consistently lose weight in a safe and progressive way. Once you start, you'll find it quite easy to juice fast for 24 hours every week.

The first 2 days are meant for preparation, while day 3 is reserved for your actual 100 percent juice fast. On days 4 and 5, you slowly return to solid food. On days 6 and 7, you're free to resume your normal eating habits, although it's highly recommended that you work your way toward a plant-based diet for long-term health benefits.

Follow this protocol once a week for a month or two, and you'll notice very impressive results in maintaining a proper body weight and exceptional health. When you reach your ideal weight, revisit this fast any time you feel the need for a quick cleanse.

Day 1:

> *Breakfast:* 16 ounces Berry Smoothie (Chapter 7)
>
> *Lunch:* Raw Nori Submarine Sandwich (Chapter 7)
>
> *Snack:* 16 ounces of any juice from Chapter 8 and No Bean Raw Hummus (Chapter 7) served with vegetable sticks
>
> *Dinner:* Avocado Boats (Chapter 7) and Raw Creamy Pea Soup (Chapter 7)

Day 2:

    Breakfast: Raw Waldorf Salad (Chapter 7)

    Lunch: Creamy Kale Soup (Chapter 7)

    Snack: 32 ounces any juice from Chapter 7 or 8, or 16 ounces Berry Smoothie (Chapter 7)

    Dinner: 32 ounces Green Smoothie (Chapter 7)

Day 3:

    Breakfast: any juice from Chapter 8

    Lunch: Celery Green Apple Spinach Juice (Chapter 10)

    Snack: Pineapple Grape Ginger Juice (Chapter 8)

    Dinner: Apple Ginger Parsley Carrot Juice (Chapter 9)

Day 4:

    Breakfast: 32 ounces Green Smoothie (Chapter 7)

    Lunch: 16 ounces Berry Smoothie (Chapter 7)

    Snack: 32 ounces of any juice from Chapter 9

    Dinner: Raw Waldorf Salad (Chapter 7)

Day 5:

    Breakfast: Green Smoothie (Chapter 7) or Berry Smoothie (Chapter 7)

    Lunch: Avocado Kale Salad (Chapter 7)

    Snack: 32 ounces of any juice from Chapter 9

    Dinner: Avocado Boats (Chapter 7) and Super Mixed Green Salad (Chapter 7)

> **TANTALIZING TIP**
>
> If it helps, think of juice fasting once a week as a healthy shift in your eating habits rather than some diet or weight-loss program. This program is not really a diet. Rather, consider it a long-term eating plan. Consuming food intermittent with fasting combines the best of many different diets without getting too restrictive. You get to enjoy the benefits of juice fasting along with enzyme-rich, easy-to-digest raw vegan meals, and should you choose, richer meals and indulgent treats on your days off. This "intermittent fasting" is the most natural way to attain long-lasting health benefits while working toward your perfect weight and well-being.

The 7-Day Slim and Sexy System

As we covered in "The 1-Day Perfect Weight-Loss Prescription," the 7-day juice fast has been expanded here to include the 2 days prior to your fast and the 2 days following breaking the fast. These are general guidelines and can be followed loosely. As a general rule, you can eat any of the recipes from Chapter 6 during the first 2 days as long as your last meal is a green smoothie or some other type of whole fruit or vegetable meal. You should also feel free to replace any of these recipes with a variety of whole fruits and vegetables or green smoothies if you prefer.

Because this is a longer fast, set aside several days to begin and end your fast for the most effective weight-loss results. You can expect to lose an average of 1 pound a day on juice-fasting days. You may drop even more as your body rids itself of any stored accumulated waste.

Day 1:

Breakfast: Raw Waldorf Salad (Chapter 7)

Lunch: Avocado Kale Salad (Chapter 7)

Snack: 16 ounces of any juice from Chapter 10, or 16 ounces Berry Smoothie (Chapter 7)

Dinner: Avocado Boats (Chapter 7) and Raw Spinach Soup (Chapter 7)

Day 2:

> *Breakfast:* 16 ounces Berry Smoothie (Chapter 7)
>
> *Lunch:* Raw Nori Submarine Sandwich (Chapter 7)
>
> *Snack:* 16 ounces of any juice from Chapter 9 or 10, or Spinach Apple Soup (Chapter 7)
>
> *Dinner:* 16 ounces Green Smoothie (Chapter 7)

Day 3:

> *Breakfast:* 32 ounces Orange Grapefruit Strawberry Juice (Chapter 8)
>
> *Lunch:* 32 ounces Cucumber Beet Carrot Juice (Chapter 9)
>
> *Snack:* 32 ounces Carrot Apple Lemon Juice (Chapter 9)
>
> *Dinner:* 32 ounces Cucumber Lemon Kale Ginger Juice (Chapter 10)

JUICY FACT

During your juice fast, you have free reign to use your intuition when it comes to what juices to drink throughout the day. We recommend juices from particular chapters to be sure you have a good balance of green building and fruit cleansing juices at all times. Ultimately, you know your preferences and the juicy concoctions you favor.

Days 4 through 9:

> *Breakfast:* 32 ounces of any juice from Chapter 8
>
> *Lunch:* 32 ounces of any juice from Chapter 9, 10, or 11
>
> *Snack:* 32 ounces of any juice from Chapter 8, 11, or 12
>
> *Dinner:* 32 ounces of any juice from Chapter 9 or 10

Day 10:

> *Breakfast:* 32 ounces Green Smoothie (Chapter 7)
>
> *Lunch:* 32 ounces of any juice from Chapter 9 or 10
>
> *Snack:* 16 or 32 ounces Berry Smoothie (Chapter 7)
>
> *Dinner:* 32 ounces Green Smoothie (Chapter 7)

Day 11:

> *Breakfast:* 16 ounces Berry Smoothie (Chapter 7)
>
> *Lunch:* 32 ounces of any juice from Chapter 9
>
> *Snack:* 16 ounces Green Smoothie (Chapter 7)
>
> *Dinner:* Avocado Kale Salad (Chapter 7)

With either of this chapter's weight loss protocols, you'll see a healthy shift in your shape after just one fast. When you revisit these fasts biweekly or monthly, you'll transform your body more quickly than you could even imagine. Feel free to make use of either of these fasts interchangeably or just stick with the one that works best for you and your lifestyle.

The Least You Need to Know

- Juice fasting is the perfect method for losing weight.
- Regular juice fasting provides the best results and keeps the weight off.
- You won't be excessively hungry while juice fasting.
- Juice fasting feeds you on a cellular level.
- Weight loss helps cleanse your body of toxins.

Juice Fasting for Cleansing

In This Chapter

- The basics of detoxification
- How to cleanse your body naturally
- Making detoxification effective and comfortable
- Possible side effects and solutions for them
- Herbs help detoxification

Your body regularly cleanses itself all the time. This is one constantly working aspect of your metabolic processes. In order to keep your body healthy and fully functioning, your cells are devoted to consistently building new tissues and their smaller component parts, repairing damaged tissues, replicating DNA, burning the energy that keeps you moving, and removing waste products from inside your cells. In fact, *cleansing* is just a fancy word for this ongoing cycle of waste removal that keeps your cells healthy and operating at their full capacity.

The problem comes when we eat diets that include heavy, rich foods that are difficult to digest. When you eat heavy protein foods and animal products, you slow your body's ability to cleanse, and eating fried foods—laden with salt and sugar—brings your cleansing processes to a complete halt. Your normal cellular respiration is stifled when those large fat molecules attach to your cell walls, preventing other nutrients from entering and waste products from leaving. This makes it difficult for cells to produce energy, and waste products start building up.

This all creates a very inhospitable condition for health, but it makes a great breeding ground for all kinds of illnesses. It's actually quite easy to create disease states in your body. All you need to do is eat processed food and animal products.

Fortunately, it's just as easy to create balance in your body. All you have to do is eat whole, plant foods. In general, nearly all plant foods are cleansing, and none contribute to toxicity in your organs or cells. Of course, if you're trying to restore your health, you may need to do more than just eat delicious fruits and veggies. You'll actually need to cleanse your body on a deeper level by detoxifying your cells with the aid of a juice fast.

What's Detoxification All About?

After your body utilizes nutrients from the food you consume, it must dispose of the unused food particles and waste products produced by digestion. If you make poor food choices, your sluggish cleansing processes can't keep up with all the toxins entering your body. They build up and accumulate rather than make their way out as they would normally. Your regular cleansing process simply doesn't have the gusto to remove all that junk. When your energy is consumed with digesting unnatural food, it just doesn't have the resources to apply toward cleansing.

Detoxification is more laborious than the regular cleansing your body tries to do on a daily basis. It's a purging of all the by-products and garbage that gets backed up and hidden away. This is an accelerated cleansing that literally takes out the trash. Your body naturally goes into detoxification mode while you sleep and when you feel inclined to eat lighter. Any time you take a break from eating, your body seizes the moment to do some deeper detoxification as damage control.

PULPY PITFALL

Your body tends to clump toxins together rather than let them permeate your entire body. This mass of dead cells allows fungal forms to reproduce and grow. It's thought that these fungal forms, in combination with the toxins that alter normal cell functioning, become the basis for malignant tumors.

Juice fasting is the ideal method for encouraging detoxification because the nutrients in fresh juice gives you energy while healing your suffering organs, suppressing disease progression, and encouraging your body to remove toxins.

You can make major improvements to your health by juice fasting and giving your body the chance to flush out all those stored-up pollutants. And after you've removed the bulk of your toxic load, your body will be quickly restored to its naturally healthy state of balance and ease. But regular detoxification is the only way to get there.

Cleansing Your Digestive System

Detoxification can happen in several ways, but generally, it begins in the digestive system. Eating fiber-rich foods like leafy greens, fruits, and other plant foods—as we recommend before you begin your juice fast—cleans out your colon and tones your entire digestive tract. This primes you for major waste removal. During the course of your juice fast, you'll notice that you continue to eliminate waste for a much longer timeframe than you might expect. You'll finally be removing the accumulated waste your body wasn't able to get rid of while eating rich foods.

You need to keep your digestive system healthy if you want to be healthy. When you don't eliminate waste properly, undigested food becomes compacted and impacted in your colon. If the surface of your bowels is covered in this way, you can't properly dispose of the normal waste products your body needs to remove on a daily basis, and you can't absorb nutrition properly. Those waste products end up being stored in your fat cells and in your organs and will eventually begin making you sick.

On the other hand, when your digestive system is working the way it was meant to, any toxins that enter your body can immediately be removed. Cleaning out your digestive system helps get you to that place where your body does what it needs to do with perfect harmony.

To totally clean out your colon and regenerate your stomach lining, you'll need to take a more proactive approach than just juice fasting alone. Daily enemas are essential when cleaning out your body.

It's also important to schedule a session for colon hydrotherapy during your cleanse. In addition, we recommend taking specific herbs to help heal, tone, and restore your intestinal lining to perfect health. If you don't choose to clean out your colon, it could take several years of juice fasting to finally remove the deeply rooted waste accumulated in your intestines.

If you really want to get the most out of your juice fasting experience, invest in the colon cleansing power of enemas and hydrotherapy, and be sure to use herbs—like the ones we recommend in our protocols— to help heal your digestive system and optimize your detoxification.

> **TANTALIZING TIP**
>
> Because digestive health is the basis for your whole body's health, it's worthwhile to utilize juice-fasting protocols and herbs that cleanse each part of your digestive tract. At one point or another, repairing your digestive health will be the only way for you to restore balance to your body.

Resetting Your Health

Detoxification is ultimately about pressing the reset button on your health. You basically get a brand-new body after you spend some time clearing out your toxic burden and restoring your organs to their intended glory. Of course, this takes more than one juice fast to achieve, but with determination and a good understanding of the causes behind disease and the forces of health, anyone can get there.

Once your digestive system is clean, you can start healing your other organs, too. They'll finally be able to remove the waste they've been bombarded with, and you can give each one some help in doing so by regular juice fasting. The longer and the more often you juice fast, the more toxic sludge you'll remove.

You can also try different protocols and herbal combinations to target the various systems in your body and get well-rounded cleansing action that repairs all your organs. It's wise to start with shorter, more basic juice fasts and work your way into more regimented fasts with accompanying herbal formulas.

Between your juice fasts, you can also drink as many fresh juices and green smoothies as you like to keep your organs working well and cleansing properly. The more you improve your diet between your juice fasts, the more effective your detoxification will be during your fasts and the more quickly you'll reset your health on every level.

Why Organic Is Essential

It's easy to say eating organic food is good for your health. At this point in the game, most of us are aware that eating conventional produce means you're also ingesting toxic and potentially lethal herbicides, pesticides, and fungicides along with petroleum-based fertilizers. Yes, organic is better. And it's absolutely essential to your cleansing process to keep these chemicals out of your body while you're in detox mode.

Juicing "conventionally" produced produce will *not* assist your cleansing process, and it's a good way to create toxicity in your body. You'd basically be pumping nutrient-rich poison into your body. This would wreak havoc on your organs and completely thwart your efforts to make your body a cleaner, more inhabitable vessel.

Keep in mind that U.S. Department of Agriculture–certified organic produce isn't completely perfect, either, which you may find surprising. Many plant-based pesticides have been cleared for use on organic produce, but none are carcinogenic or toxic in the way their commercially produced counterparts are. If you want the best of the best, try to get your produce from growers who don't spray at all.

Your best bet for high-quality produce may, in fact, be your local organic farms and farmers' markets. If you live in an area where local organic produce is hard to come by, you can always order bulk produce from online retailers or encourage your local grocery store to stock more organic produce. If they're not so hip to the idea of increasing their organic produce department, see if they're willing to order bulk cases of fruits and vegetables for you during your cleanse. Yes, *cases*. You'll easily go through a case of apples during a week-long juice fast!

What to Expect While Cleansing

Just knowing what you might run into before starting a juice fast can help you mentally prepare for anything that might come up emotionally or physically during a detox. Sometimes being caught unaware is enough to thwart your efforts. If you're not sure why you're suddenly having a hard time, it can be very disconcerting.

Your first juice fast might be a challenge. You might feel constantly tempted to break your fast and eat different kinds of food rather than see it through to the end. When you stop putting addictive substances (even things like sugar and salt are addictive) into your body, you go through a withdrawal.

After you get through the first 3 days or so of a cleanse, you should notice that you actually have tons of energy, your urge to eat subsides, and you feel great in general. This is especially true of shorter cleanses. They tend to give your body enough of a cleanse that you feel really good each time you do one.

A longer juice fast encourages deeper detoxification, and your experience on a juice fast lasting longer than a week could prove drastically different from your previous shorter juice fasts. After a week of juice fasting, your body really starts flushing out the toxins stored in your tissues. With them can come all kinds of strange and uncomfortable symptoms. This is often referred to as a healing crises. It may mirror a severe cold or flu, but the symptoms don't last nearly as long.

Even though these other symptoms can be inconvenient or unpleasant, they're a sign your body is utilizing this time to do some serious deep-cleaning. This happens because as toxins are flushed from your tissues, they reenter your bloodstream and filter through your organs for removal. Any time you have toxins filtering through your body, you'll feel ill. It's actually normal and safe to let these adversities play out, but you can certainly help your body do its job more efficiently by trying some of the adjunct treatments suggested in this chapter and in Chapter 4.

After a period of deep detox, most people find themselves in a very euphoric state of awareness. You may have elaborate dreams you remember easily upon awakening, and you could likely encounter a deep state of loving acceptance stemming from the permeating calm you feel inside. You may encounter profound feelings that everything in your world is just right and start enjoying being in the moment. Your intuition will become finely tuned, and you may begin to understand things about yourself and those around you that you'd overlooked before.

JUICY FACT

When you feel light and clean in your body and your mind feels sharp and calm, you naturally become euphoric. You may find yourself looking forward to your next juice fast just to get that feeling back.

Possible Detox Symptoms

While some of the more pleasant side effects of detoxification may include clearer skin, restful sleep, and a decrease in disease symptoms, you may also experience uncomfortable side effects. Some of the more common ones include night sweats, hot and cold flashes, chills, headaches, a runny nose, fatigue, body aches, and other general flulike symptoms. You may also have very drastically varied energy levels throughout the day. These things can happen sporadically and will vary in intensity according to the amount of toxic buildup being removed and by how efficiently you remove it.

These symptoms may come on very quickly and can leave quickly as well. You might feel fine one morning only to find yourself completely overcome with fatigue all of a sudden. Sometimes these symptoms may need to play out for a few days just like a regular flu, and other times they may seem to miraculously disappear before you even notice it. So don't worry about spending an entire month-long juice fast in misery. That just won't happen.

When you detox at a deep level, you might experience symptoms of the health issues you've had throughout your life in reverse as they leave your body. So if you've recently had problems with arthritis, you may notice that after being relieved for some time, your symptoms suddenly flare up again. Keep going on your juice fast until they disappear. They will!

If you've done several juice fasts already, you may notice that each one brings out different symptoms. All of a sudden you may start to feel the expression of childhood asthma or earaches begin to manifest, but these, too, will quickly resolve.

These symptoms are a sign your body is doing its job and getting those toxins out for good, but there are many things you can do to speed the process along or slow down your detoxification a bit to a level that's more comfortable for you. After all, it might be very inconvenient for you to suddenly encounter a terrible headache while you're trying to work.

Optimizing Your Body

As mentioned earlier, the first thing most people notice when they start cleaning out their bodies is an increase in their energy levels. This happens when your cells are relieved of the burden of removing excess waste products in addition to the normal by-products of cellular respiration. Then they can devote more time to converting complex nutrients into *ATP* and using it as fuel to create energy for your entire body.

DEFINITION

ATP, or **adenosine triphosphate,** is a molecule found in all living cells and is used for all biological processes that require energy. It's most easily manufactured by breaking down simple and complex sugars into the component molecules needed to recharge your body.

When your body is so clean you can feel the tingling sensation of life pulsating through your cells, you'll feel as if you've been reborn. You'll develop a relationship with your body you never knew was possible. It will communicate with you through sensations, strong urges, and a deep sense of understanding. It will tell you how to feed it and when. You won't have to ponder in confusion over mysterious symptoms or relinquish your youth to the ills of aging.

In a way, you're going through a rebirth of a sort. When your tissues completely regenerate and your DNA is fully activated, your entire body and being will be completely different from the former version of yourself. No longer subject to genetic predispositions or chemical imbalances, your electrified brainpower and virile body will become the perfect tools for creating a happy, long, and successful life.

Supporting Healthy Detoxification

To support your healthy detoxification while keeping it from taking over your life, you should enlist the help of a few adjunct therapies. An enema or colonic can eradicate detox head and body aches. You can also try taking a bentonite clay supplement to help move the toxins out of your body. Enlist the aid of some powerful herbs to deepen your detox and heal your organs, too.

We highly recommend you take a bit of zeolite in either a powdered clay form or a suspended liquid every day during your cleanse, particularly on fasts lasting longer than 7 days. Zeolites are a class of minerals known as molecular sieves. They basically absorb any positively charged molecules in the order of their size, from largest to smallest. When you ingest them, they attract and trap heavy metals like mercury and strontium 90, chemicals like formaldehyde and freon, and even microscopic parasites and viruses! Regularly taking zeolites can do wonders for cleaning your body and helps ensure you don't reabsorb the toxins being flushed from your tissues during your juice fast.

JUICY FACT

Zeolites absorb positively charged free radicals into their hollow, honeycomb-shape structure. Once this mineral absorbs a toxic substance, it can no longer come into direct contact with your tissues and won't be hanging around making you sick—even if it's not immediately removed from your body.

Getting your blood and lymph system moving are another great way to support healthy detoxification. When your blood vessels dilate, they become more permeable. Toxins can more easily move from your tissues into your bloodstream and then into your lymph system for removal through your elimination organs.

To support healthy detoxification, you'll need to either deepen your detox or soften it a bit to ensure you're removing the waste without letting it make you sick. Mild detox symptoms are fine, but you don't want them to become so intense they take over your life and make you really ill. In fact, if you do feel ill, you may be reabsorbing toxins rather than removing them.

The Key to True Detoxification

It might be surprising to know that the key to deep detoxification during your juice fast is getting regular colon hydrotherapy. You should do a daily enema at home or schedule weekly colonics by a professional hydrotherapist any time you juice fast for a week or more.

Fresh juices are incredibly detoxifying on their own, and when you add herbs that push your detox deeper, you end up with an abundance of toxins circulating in your body fighting to be removed. But juices lack the fibrous bulk that helps push waste products out of your body. You can add psyllium husks or chia seeds to your juices for increased bulk that will help remove that stuff, but ultimately, enemas and colonics are the most effective method for clearing out the impacted fecal matter that lingers in nearly everyone's digestive system. A good cleaning out can cure you of detox symptoms such as headaches during your cleanse.

Juicing does give you some fiber though, and will certainly purify and cleanse your bowels, but the process is much slower. Many of us simply can't afford to wait around for our bodies to get that stuff out on their own. If you have health issues, you need to clear out your colon now so you can start detoxing the substances making you ill. Even if you're not sick, why would you want to wait around for a life-changing shift in the way you look and feel? Getting a colonic during your juice fast can do this for you almost instantly, and you'll be flushing out those old pollutants in no time!

Colonics are also the most efficient way to prevent and clear up detox symptoms. This is true while you're juice fasting, and it also applies to any other area of your life. If you're sick with a fever or a cough you just can't kick due to the flu season or a cleansing juice fast, getting a colonic will immediately halt your symptoms.

Doing a daily enema during your juice fast can do wonders for keeping your blood and body clean as you detox, but at some point you should also do a colonic because the volume of water used is far greater, meaning deeper cleansing, resulting in incredible health benefits.

Helpful Herbs

At this point, we're sure you've gotten the message that plant foods are healthy and healing, but it's important to note that certain plants, not normally used for food, have potent healing abilities when taken in small amounts. These are collectively called herbs, but this umbrella term also includes certain fungi, seaweeds, algae, fruits, and spices in addition to the familiar, pungent, leafy greens we use to season our food. There are tons of uses for these various herbs, and many have great synergistic compatibilities.

Each herb comes with a different set of phytochemicals that have powerful actions in your body. Because of this, it's important to use our recommendations as a general guideline and use the herbs that are best for you. You can let intuition be your guide while experimenting with various herbs, or you can find professional rec-ommendations and see how they work for you.

You can use a number of herbs during your juice fast to deepen your detoxification. These herbs open your circulatory system, flush your kidneys, and detox your liver or colon. Countless others have been cited for their ability to shrink malignant tumors, and many others are reputed with being able to eradicate cancer cells altogether.

Many herbs are helpful because they're considered *adaptogens*. They can be useful for a variety of ailments and include many mild herbs that can be safely taken by adults as well as children. These herbs give you an energy boost during your fast and help build your immunity.

DEFINITION

Adaptogens give your body nonspecific immunity to diseases. They help balance the endocrine system and strengthen weak tissues.

Herbs can be incredibly helpful and healing for digestive disorders. Even though digestive health is easily disturbed with the wrong type of food, its tissues are also one of the easiest to regenerate. The stomach lining can regenerate in just 2 days, and the intestines can regenerate in 4 days! With the help of a few soothing herbs, your juice fast can do miraculous things for your digestive health.

Even though fungi aren't members of the plant kingdom, we include them in the "herb" category for their tonic and healing abilities. A few very special mushrooms contain the most potent disease-fighting phytochemicals of any herb or plant of the fungus kingdom. They're all very synergistic and can be taken together with no ill effect. Some medicinal mushrooms to consider taking are reishi, shiitake, lion's mane, maitake, tremella, poria, turkey tail, himematsutake, and zhu ling.

Don't underestimate the power of common herbs. Peppermint, thyme, oregano, lavender, rosemary, black pepper, lemongrass, and many other cooking herbs are also incredibly healing and detoxifying.

Alleviating Symptoms

If you're really having intense detox symptoms you can't handle or feel like they're more detrimental than helpful to your cleanse, there are several things you can do to resolve the situation. The first thing to do is add 2 or 3 tablespoons chia seeds into your next juice. Just be sure to stir the combination well and let it sit for at least 10 minutes to let the chia seeds gel. This gel is incredibly nutritious and is very healing to your digestive system. It helps absorb the toxins and adds enough bulk to push them out of your body.

JUICY FACT

The chia seed has been used by the Tarahumara people of northwestern Mexico to provide lasting energy on 100-mile runs. It's said that just 1 or 2 tablespoons can help an athlete sustain this kind of physical exertion for an entire day.

Another symptom reducer, as mentioned, is a colonic. Do your best to schedule one as soon as possible or invest in a home enema kit. This gives you almost immediate relief. Take some zeolite or bentonite to help absorb those toxins, too.

You can also soak in hot water, sunbathe, or do some moderate exercise. Exercise might seem like the last thing you want to do when you don't feel well, but it will help you sweat out the toxins.

If the juice fast feels too intense for you, one option to slow things down is a switch to green smoothies instead of juices for a serving. Replace one of your regularly scheduled juices with a green smoothie and then return to your juicing program later in the day. You could also drink green smoothies for several days and then pick up the juice fast when it feels more manageable. This way you'll still be cleansing even though your detoxification slows down.

Take your body's cues seriously. You might have to dig deep to figure out if you're just dealing with cravings or attachments to food, or if you're actually going through detox. The last thing you need to do is feel stressed out during your juice fast, so ease back on it if you need to and then dive back in when you're ready.

The Least You Need to Know

- Detoxification is a natural process of accelerated cleansing.
- Your digestive health is the keystone to the health of your whole body.
- Organic produce is essential to your cleansing process.
- Detoxification can cause uncomfortable symptoms, but many therapies can minimize these cleansing reactions.
- Colon hydrotherapy ensures proper and complete removal of toxins.
- Herbs can aid your detox process and heal your organs.

Getting the Most from Your Juice Fast

In This Chapter

- Fitting a juice fast into your schedule
- Including family and friends in your fast
- Beginning a juice fast properly
- The importance of ending a fast well

You're probably excited to jump right in to your first juice fast. But wait just a moment. To reap the full benefits and safely perform a juice fast, there's some important information you need to know before diving in.

As you learned in Chapter 3, a juice fast is a powerful method for ridding your body of accumulated toxins caused by unhealthy foods, environmental pollutants, and metabolic by-products. But unless you follow the right protocol and find yourself a supportive environment, you can cause more stress on your body than if you skipped the fast altogether.

By using one of the many protocols we've mapped out in this book, you can properly prepare yourself for getting the most out of your fast. We highly recommend that you follow our advice for the preparation phase—and even more importantly, ending your fast—as outlined in this chapter.

Working Juice Fasting into Your Life

The nice thing about juice fasting is that you can easily adapt a program to suit your individual needs. You can either make your juice fast work around your life or adapt your life to work around your juice fast. It's important to remember that you can experience a wide range of emotions and energy levels during your fast, so choosing a good time to do it is very important to your success.

As we mentioned in previous chapters, you should feel free to experiment, slowly, while getting ready for your first juice fast. Rather than jumping into a fast, you can try replacing a meal here and there with a fresh juice. Then when you're feeling more comfortable with the process and juicing in general, you can graduate to a short 1- or 3-day juice fast.

Use your juice fasts as a mark of forward motion toward your health goals. It really is the perfect way to catapult yourself toward better eating habits. Each time you break your fast, you'll be motivated to maintain your high energy levels and sexy, trim waistline by eating healthy, whole, plant-based foods. Use this to your advantage!

You can do a longer juice fast as part of a major overhaul on your entire life and eating habits, or you can do a series of shorter fasts while making small changes to your basic eating habits each time. Making small changes to your diet by eliminating one or two types of unhealthy food each time you fast is a realistic, low-pressure method for cleaning up your diet and consistently improving your health. There's really no need to do it all at once, unless you're in the middle of a healing crisis, and a gradual change is more likely to be a long-lasting one.

After you end your fast, you'll want to integrate juicing into your daily routine. If you're trying to lose weight, you might even consider replacing one of your daily meals with a fresh juice. This way, you'll still be encouraging continuous weight loss between your juice fasts and packing in some super nutrition at the same time.

Scheduling Your Juice Fast

You may be wondering how to go about choosing a "good time" to juice fast. Naturally, this depends on the people you'll be around and the places you'll spend your time. Take inventory of the social situations that make you feel at ease and relaxed as opposed to those that create tension or overexcitement. You'll have to decide for yourself what you can handle and what would be an ideal or acceptable environment to fast in. Then you can make an educated decision about choosing a time that best fits your needs and your life.

It can be wonderful to have friends and family around while juice fasting. You might find that many people are interested in your motivation for going on a fast and may even ask you for advice about their own health. On the other hand, not everyone understands health and the process of healing enough to appreciate your efforts, and some may criticize you or try to dissuade you from your cleanse. If you'd like to avoid such unwanted scrutiny, it might be best to fast on days when you know you won't be around people who stir up negative emotions or cause excessive stress in your life.

For example, many people decide to do a short cleanse over the weekend, but if you live in a house that has hectic weekends full of chores and shuttling your family around to various activities, it might be easier for you to try juice fasting during the week, even if you work.

TANTALIZING TIP

Drinking upward of a quart of juice or more means you may need to use the bathroom more frequently than usual. Just be sure your boss understands you may need more breaks during the week you fast so you don't draw too much attention to the fact.

Lots of people find it quite easy and enjoyable to fast discreetly during the workweek, and this is something we've had great success doing ourselves. Fasting while going about your daily life can actually be much easier than you might expect. As long as you enjoy your job and it doesn't feel too stressful, you can continue your normal activities regardless of your juice fast. If you're planning on doing a fast for a week or more and can't take time off from work, it'll be necessary that your fast coincide with work at some point.

It's helpful that juicers come in all shapes and sizes, and fortunately, some of the best ones are also small and easily portable. If you're planning to juice fast during your workweek, consider checking ahead to see if you can take your juicer along to work and set it up in the break room. This way you can make fresh juices during your normal lunch break or during another convenient time. And if that's not an option, you could always prepare a couple quarts of juice before work to bring along with you. Whatever makes the process easy and hassle free is going to work best.

If you're just not into juice fasting while you work or if you have a high-stress job, you might need to take a weekend at home or even a solo jaunt out on your own to get the space you need to feel great during your juice fast. And if you're planning on doing a long juice fast of 28 days or longer, explore your options for taking some time off of work to juice fast at home or at a retreat center.

Don't feel guilty if you need to take some space from your family or friends to get some deep rest and healing. The people who love you want you to feel your best, and they'll be happy to have you come home enlivened and feeling great.

Mentally Preparing Yourself

The process of juice fasting is about more than the fast itself. It's an entire cleansing regimen that integrates the days surrounding the juice fast into the detoxification process. You'll be better off if you automatically assume that a 1-day juice fast will actually be a 4- or 5-day cleanse. This way, when you decide to embark on a juice fast, you'll be mentally prepared. We cannot stress how important it is to end your fast slowly, with determined integrity.

Over the course of a fast lasting a week or more, you can certainly expect to have drastically changing energy levels and possibly mood swings or some of the other detox symptoms discussed in Chapter 3. Each fast may be slightly different from the last. Chances are you'll get through your first couple juice fasts and experience nothing but tons of energy while feeling great the entire time. Then you might find that a later fast brings out flulike symptoms. In general, shorter fasts make you feel rejuvenated while longer fasts may take you through some more intense ups and downs. These symptoms are nothing to worry about, but it's good to know ahead of time that you might have some of this stuff come up.

Don't be surprised if at times you feel emotional during your fast. This might not bother you, but for some people, handling bouts of intense emotions, particularly while they're working, can be hard to cope with. Just take a break if you find yourself in this position. Go out for some air and do some deep breathing. You can also pull back the cleansing process by drinking more vegetable juices and less fruit juices or using some of the suggestions on this topic from Chapter 3.

Cravings are another thing you might encounter while you fast. This is particularly true during the first 3 days. Unless you're a seasoned juice faster, don't expect to go the entire time without having a craving or two sneak up on you. Just take a drink of juice or water, and think about how much better your body feels when you drink a fresh juice instead of reaching for unhealthy food.

PULPY PITFALL

You may crave certain foods during your juice fast and be very tempted to break your fast and eat. Please don't! Cravings come because your body is releasing toxic substances from leftover components of comfort foods. Do not eat comfort foods before your juice fast is over or use them to break your fast, or you can cause serious damage to your body.

Fortunately, cravings subside after a few days and are unlikely to return. If you do have cravings after this period of time while on a longer juice fast, they'll be far less intense and more manageable than the initial cravings. The longer you juice fast, the easier it becomes because your body starts to sense what it wants and needs. If you explore how you feel while having a craving, you might be surprised to find that the food you think you're craving actually seems repulsive when you consider eating it!

You may need to rest while you're fasting. A desk job may let you catch your breath while still being productive, but there's always a chance you'll just need to sleep while you fast. Plan for this in advance if you can, but don't hesitate to take the time to care for your needs if they come up in a way that surprises you. Leave work for the day if you need to—you can always cut your fast short and bump up your break-fast protocol if the fast is interfering with your obligations.

If you do decide to cut a fast short, consider stretching out your transition diet for several days more than what we recommended. You don't need to limit yourself to drinking smoothies for a week after your fast, but it wouldn't hurt to stick to a simple raw vegan diet for as long as you like afterward. An enzyme-rich diet full of minerals and phytonutrients can do wonders for your ongoing health maintenance. This also helps you continue cleansing in a milder way, and you'll already be prepared if you want to pick up the fast again on the weekend.

Keep in mind that staying positive and maintaining a good attitude during a juice fast is essential. The information we've offered here about some possible troubles during your cleanse are not guaranteed to happen to you, so don't go into your fast expecting to feel terrible or have a difficult time staying away from the foods you like. Just be open to whatever the fast brings. Each time can be different, and it's entirely possible for you to enjoy the process regardless of what comes up.

JUICY FACT

When you prioritize a positive attitude, you automatically increase your longevity, increase your immunity, and reduce your risk of a host of diseases. Plus, you find the strength to power through bouts of depression!

Creating a Support Network

For many of us, having a support network turns a challenge like juice fasting for the first time into an infinitely more enjoyable experience. Sometimes just knowing you can talk to someone about the hard parts of your fast, as well as the parts that exhilarate you, can be exactly what you need to make the juice-fasting process a complete success!

It can also be wonderfully supportive and bonding to juice fast with a buddy. Your fasting buddy could be any enthusiastic person you know—your significant other, a good friend, a work colleague, a family member, or even an online juice-fasting group. Being able to discuss your milestones and hardships with someone who understands and has been there can empower you to keep going. It can make the difference in whether or not you follow through with a long-term fast or encourage you to start one for the first time. A fasting partner can gently help hold you accountable to your intentions and keep you from sliding back into old habits and is someone you can hang out with when you feel out of sync with the other people in your life.

This person is also someone you can celebrate with! It's one thing to be an army of one on the road to health and self-improvement, but it makes a world of difference to have company on this sometimes-lonely path. There's nothing like going to a social event and being the only one refraining from party food, but if you have your fasting buddy at your side, the two of you may just become the topic of interest at the gathering! Plus, when you both complete your fasts, you can continue to support one another by making healthy food together and keeping each other on track toward your individual goals.

Maybe you can't find a fasting buddy this time around, but if you're lucky enough to have understanding and supportive friends or family members, include them in your cleanse even if they're not partaking. Talk to your people ahead of time, and ask them if it's okay to call them when you need support. That way you can call them for pep talks if you come upon a moment of weakness or feel tempted to eat something you know you shouldn't. You can always entice them to come listen to your woes by offering to make them some of the most delicious juice they'll ever taste!

There are other ways to enlist the help of others and create a supportive surrounding, too. Suppose you're responsible for most of the cooking in your household; it might be wise to set a menu ahead of time for any family members who aren't joining you on your juice fast. This way, you don't have to spend tons of time thinking about food. You could make a few meals ahead of time and freeze them or enlist the help of someone else to take over these duties while you take a break and focus on your juicing.

> **TANTALIZING TIP**
>
> Juice fasting by yourself when everyone else in your house is eating their favorite foods could be difficult. To combat this pitfall, enlist the help of your family to support you during your cleanse. You can ask them to make juice with you or give them a glass to drink along with their meal. You can let them know you won't be around for mealtime for a few days while you drink your juices in a restful, private place away from the bustle and temptation of the family table.

Another way to keep your entire family involved is to encourage them to eat a modified version of your juice fast, if they're open to it. You could serve them simple blended meals like smoothies and raw soups that are a cinch to make rather than laboriously pour over a hot stove. Everyone in your house will be improving their health, and tempting foods will stay out of your home.

If your family isn't keen on the idea of eating a modified diet while you juice fast, and you just don't feel like you can make normal meals for your family while juice fasting, tell them you'll be taking a break from meal-making for the duration of your fast, and relinquish the task to another available family member. The person who has to pick up the slack may feel reluctant or may enthusiastically offer to help, but either way, convey to this family member that a healthy you is better able to care for the family so your healing time needs to be a priority.

Planning a juice fast that supports you and those around you may seem like a difficult task to take on if you're doing it alone. That's why keeping those around you informed and involved in any way you can is ultimately a recipe for success. And don't hesitate to let your support network know how much you appreciate their love and understanding.

Sharing Your Juice!

Every time you make juice, you create an opportunity to turn on someone else to the amazing benefits of juicing and juice fasting. As long as you feel inclined to offer, most people would love to partake in your bounty of fresh juices. This small gesture alone could be enough to set someone on their own journey to health and vitality, so don't be shy about sharing.

In fact, this can be an ideal way to include your family members and even your friends in your juice fast. Give your kids their own glass of the juice you're drinking for breakfast, and offer more in the afternoon as part of a healthy snack. Nearly all kids love juice, and you'll be doing them a favor by replacing any of their pasteurized, nutritionally bankrupt juices with fresh ones. Helping kids see that they love fresh juices can create a lifetime of healthy eating habits!

If your kids are drinking juices and enjoying them, take the opportunity to use their enthusiasm to fuel your own during your juice fast. If you need some extra motivation to get going and press that first juice for the morning, let your kids' watering mouths be that motivation! You can even let older kids make your juice for you while you relax. Now how's that for service?

> **TANTALIZING TIP**
>
> Let your kids be as involved in your juice fast as they want. Most kids like to help their parents in the kitchen. They may be too young to fast with you, but that doesn't mean they can't make and enjoy fresh juices with you.

When your juice fast extends into the workweek, it's very likely you'll get some questions from curious co-workers. They may wonder why you don't want to go out to lunch like usual, or they may notice you juicing in the break room. If you enjoy inspiring others, let them know what you're up to. You can offer to pour them a glass if you happened to bring along enough to share, or silently leave behind a few little cups of juice for others to find—we all know how much people love samples. That way they can take it upon themselves to try it out without feeling obligated.

Another fun way to share your juice is to make an event of it. Invite friends to a juice cocktail party during your fast so you can continue your cleanse and still enjoy the company of friends. You can set out several pitchers of different juices and serve them to your friends in fancy wine or champagne glasses. This adds an enticing element to the presentation of your juices that lets the beautiful colors be appreciated in their full glory.

If you're really feeling outgoing and enjoy entertaining, you could make your cocktail party a more regular event. You could invite your friends to pop by after work during the week for a daily juice cocktail hour for the duration of your fast. You never know, this might just be a great way for you to find the perfect juicing buddy for your next juice fast!

Making the Perfect Juice

It's a good idea to consume a wide variety of juices while you're fasting. Juice fasting may present a huge diversion from the routine of your normal life, but this process should still be easy, fun, and pleasant. Most importantly, you should always enjoy the taste of your fresh juice and try different ones regularly to keep your taste buds interested, as well as to cover all your nutritional bases. But keep in mind, you would also receive benefits from drinking the juice of even just one kind of fruit, such as grapes or melon. This is called mono juice-fasting, and many people have reversed disease following this kind of protocol as well.

Most of the juice recipes in this book were formulated with appealing flavor combinations in mind. The vast majority of our juices are sweet and very tasty. We've also included some more potent juice recipes that contain powerfully healing plants and may have slightly stronger flavors but are still quite enjoyable. Some of these plants may taste bitter, sour, or astringent on their own, but we've gone to great efforts to make the juices that contain such ingredients extremely palatable and tasty.

JUICY FACT

Bitter and astringent herbs usually indicate that they're rich in healing phytochemicals. Many plants taste bitter as a deterrent to foragers, but if you can get past the taste, they hold powerful medicinal properties.

It's actually very easy to make a potent, healing juice by pressing any number of immune-stimulating herbs, spices, fruits, veggies, and greens through your juicer. Getting the taste just right may take some trial and error though. Making the perfect juice is an experiment in alchemy. It entails delicately balancing the flavors of various ingredients so you get a delicious, mouthwatering juice with tons of life-giving nutrients and healing properties.

It takes experience, know-how, and a sense of adventure to concoct the perfect juice, and we're happy to give you a head start in the right direction. Flavor balancing can be very personal, so it's important to know if you prefer sweet to savory or sour to spicy. The recipes in this book are formulated so they'll appeal to just about anyone, but you can always use them as templates for finding exactly the right juices tailored just for you.

As you like, you can add more sweet ingredients to your juices like apples and carrots, more watery neutral ingredients like cucumber and celery, or more potent healing greens, herbs, and tonic ingredients. If ever you find that you don't jibe with the taste of a particular juice, just add a bit of apple or cucumber or even a squeeze of lemon.

Use your intuition during your juice fast. You'll feel connected and drawn to certain fruits and vegetables, so find the juices you gravitate toward and make them your own special concoctions. We've provided you with ample recipes in this book, but we also encourage you to think outside the box and create your own mixtures. As you become more intuitive and creative throughout a juice fast; you might just find that you naturally develop a sense of juice combining, too. In fact, that's how we came up with most of the juice recipes in this book.

So don't be afraid to let *your* intuition guide you and go out on a limb with some of your juice combinations. Take your favorite fruit salad ingredients or your favorite nonsweet fruits and vegetables and see what you can come up with. Chances are, your juice will taste great and be just what your body needs at that moment.

Choosing the Perfect Juicer

Store-bought pasteurized and bottled juices don't have the living enzymes, vigor, or vitamin and phytonutrient content fresh juices contain. They won't offer the same healing properties fresh juices have in abundance. It's for this reason that you should only drink fresh juices during your juice fast. If you're going to be making enough fresh juice to keep your body hydrated and nourished during your cleanse, it's important to have a high-quality juicer on hand to make this process easy.

There are many juicers on the market that range from centrifugal juicers to wheatgrass presses. We think the best all-purpose machines for juice fasting are low-rpm (rotations per minute) *single-* or *double-auger juicers* or *grind juicers*. These types of juicers protect the valuable nutrients in your fresh juice from oxidation.

DEFINITION

Both **single-** and **double-auger juicers** utilize one or two augers, the long moving piece that resembles a drill bit, to crush produce and press the juice out of the pulp as it passes over a fine screen. The **grind juicer** actually grabs the fruits and veggies and grinds them inside the hopper. This process extracts all the nutrients slowly and powerfully at the same time, maintaining more of the juice's integrity by exposing it to less oxidation than other juicers.

Another great benefit to these types of juicers is that they can press nearly anything. Many juicers on the market only have a single function—such as the wheatgrass juicer—and others won't juice greens effectively at all. They're also fairly easy to clean because you don't have to deal with a large screen or hard-to-reach crevices. They're easy to take apart and reassemble quickly. Plus, you can simply dismantle your juicer and toss the parts into the dishwasher to sterilize it regularly.

Blending Your Juice

If you haven't yet invested in a high-quality low-rpm juicer, you may still be able to enjoy the benefits of juicing. You can blend the ingredients of your chosen juice and then strain out the pulp with a piece of cheesecloth, a nut milk bag, a paint-straining bag from a hardware store, or a piece of organic muslin cloth. (You can save the pulp in the freezer and make some raw crackers or other treats with it, or discard it as you see fit.) This will give you a fresh, pulp-free juice.

If you choose to create your juices using a blender, you'll get the best results using a high-speed blender because you can include an entire recipe's worth of ingredients all at once. However, any of our recipes can be modified to suit any type of blender. If you have a standard-speed blender, you'll have to blend your juice in stages to get the best results.

Start by adding any citrus juice, if applicable, and then add softer or more water-rich fruits or vegetables like finely chopped apples or cucumber. If your blender overheats easily, you should strain this first run of blended ingredients before adding harder vegetables like beets and carrots. That way, you'll have a watery base that will aid your blender in processing harder produce. In a stronger blender, you can just liquefy your apples, cucumber, or celery and then add in carrots or other harder vegetables, finishing with any greens you plan to include. Rather than strain and return your juice to the blender—as is the case with blenders that easily overheat—before proceeding to the next ingredient, you can just strain it all at the end.

You should also halve your recipe before you begin. This helps preserve the integrity of your juice and ensures your blender stays in good working order. We prefer using a low-rpm juicer during a juice fast. If budget is an issue, you can usually pick up a used juicer quite affordably on auction-based websites. (See Appendix B for leads on used juicers.)

PULPY PITFALL

Compared to high-speed blenders, many standard blenders have a small capacity, meaning you can't squeeze a whole recipe's worth of ingredients into it at once. Even standard blenders that come with a large carafe may overheat if you fill them too full. It's best to err on the side of caution and put into your blender only what it can handle.

Beginning Your Juice Fast

So now that you know how to set yourself up for a successful juice fast, how do you actually begin it? The way you prepare your body for your juice fast greatly determines the benefit you get out of the fast itself. It's simply not wise to eat a heavy, rich, or fatty meal one day and then jump straight into a juice fast the next. You might feel better for the moment, but it won't do much for your long-term health. It's hard on your body to juice fast before giving your digestive system a mild cleanse first. You're juice fasting to relieve and cleanse your body, not cause it extra stress or damage.

We always recommend you begin by eating lighter for at least 2 days before you start a juice fast. Easing your body into a fast prepares your system for cleansing and makes even a 1-day juice fast far more effective.

First, eliminate all animal products, including dairy, plus caffeine, heavily processed foods, or overcooked food. Over the next 2 days, you'll transition toward a diet of salads, smoothies, blended raw soups, and lots of fruit. This starts the cleansing process and prepares your body to receive your fast well. As soon as you modify your diet to these healthy suggestions, your stomach will almost instantly realize it's being allowed to finally get some needed rest. This transition period also helps you psychologically, softening the dramatic shift between eating solid food and drinking only liquids.

TANTALIZING TIP

Most of us have some sort of food addiction—otherwise, it would be easy for us to eat healthfully all the time. Weaning yourself off these foods may be difficult enough before removing solid food completely. It can be hard to juice fast for the first time, especially if you don't take the time to eat lightly for a few days. Eating raw vegan foods before your juice fast gives you the comfort of solid food while you pull away from the foods you feel attached to. This greatly increases the likelihood of successful juice fasting and makes the process more enjoyable.

At this point, you may notice you already feel lighter and healthier just from switching to a diet of solid raw vegan foods. It can actually be very helpful to try using this modified diet as a periodic fast before you approach juice fasting. While juice fasting works better, faster, and more efficiently for cleansing your body, we also recommend the occasional raw vegan cleanse as a great way to diminish the difficult challenges that can come along with juice fasting and as a way to continue detoxification between juice fasts. If you're interested in completing a raw-food detox program, we recommend *The Complete Idiot's Guide to Raw Food Detox* by Adam Graham.

To plan your fast well, you need to allow for transition time before you switch to consuming strictly juices. As you allow your body to slowly shift from its normal digestive duties into cleansing mode, you'll start to clean out your colon and prevent toxins from being reabsorbed while you juice fast. Taking a couple days to eat energetic and fiber-filled raw foods tones your whole digestive tract and cleans you out so your body is primed to release excess weight and flush out unhealthy substances. This is essentially the best way to start any cleansing process, and juice fasting is no exception.

During the 2 or 3 days prior to your juice fast, you can use the recipes we offer in Chapter 7, choose mono-meals of one type of fresh fruit or vegetable, or create your own simple blended foods. With these options, you'll be doing an enormous amount of good for your digestive system and preparing yourself to receive the incredible benefits a juice fast has to offer!

The *Only* Way to End Your Juice Fast

Why would you juice fast at all if you didn't think you'd get some serious lasting benefits out of it? Right? Now that we agree on that point, let's discuss how to make your newfound level of health the platform from which you launch yourself into even *better* health!

When you're ready to end your juice fast and make the shift back toward more normal, healthy eating habits, follow the protocols outlined in this book. Ending your juice fast with the right foods is just as essential to the success of your fast as the fast itself!

Before you can resume your normal eating habits, you need to eat simply for a few days, just as you did before starting the fast. This is an essential step in the completion of your fast because it prevents the shock that can happen if you immediately overload your body with heavy or fatty foods. Your body won't be ready to break down such foods after its hiatus from solids, so you have to use caution with what and how you break your juice fast.

We cannot stress enough that you must ease out of your juice fast *slowly*. There are many reasons for this, but most important is that you don't want to shock your body with fats that make your metabolism sluggish or complex foods that are difficult to process. These foods will shut down your digestive system.

Ending your fast with simple foods that nourish without burdening your digestive system supports your cleansing processes while you return to eating whole foods. This is an ideal intermediary step because blasting your system out of cleansing mode with unhealthy food choices can make you feel sicker than you were before you started your fast. You might have a relapse back into some painful symptoms that were alleviated by the juice fast, or you may feel queasy, heavy, and toxic. Either way, the results are unanimously negative if you break your fast the wrong way.

During a juice fast, your body is in a resting and repairing state, which is similar to a partial hibernation. Eating a slice of pizza or even a bowl of brown rice directly following your fast is like walking out of a vacation in paradise and directly into a 12-hour shift at the hardest job you can imagine without sleep or any kind of transition time. Likewise, such a sudden return to a normal solid food diet can be damaging and dangerous, especially if your normal diet includes animal products. You might end up feeling incredibly ill from a poor food choice after a fast, or your body might actually reject the food you've eaten and purge it.

The simple way to avoid this is to follow our recommendations for breaking a fast. This way, you'll preserve the benefits of your juice fast and avoid becoming ill directly after.

Throughout every protocol in this book, we recommend you eat easy-to-digest, raw fruits and vegetables for at least 2 days before trying to resume normal, *healthy* eating habits. The first day after your fast should start with very simple, liquefied foods like green smoothies or blended fruits, which give your digestive system the signal it's time to resume eating solids. These types of food are basically juices with the fiber added in, and they help give your body time to switch gears slowly from resting mode to active digestive duty.

TANTALIZING TIP

The good news is for the most part, the foods you should avoid directly after your juice fast are the same foods you should try avoiding altogether. Juice fasting helps your body acclimate to a healthy diet, and as you cleanse, you'll notice your cravings for unhealthful foods fade. You'll actually start craving healthful foods, and your newly discovered intuition will communicate this to you in every way.

Later that day, you can try eating a few pieces of whole fruit of your choice. Some great choices for your first few meals are red grapes, soaked prunes, papaya, melons of all kinds, pears, cucumbers, or peaches and nectarines. These first few meals should be mono-meals unless you want to add some greens to your blended fruit. You can eat as much of this one type of fruit as you desire. Continue the day with more fruit smoothies, whole fruit, or juices whenever you feel hungry.

During the second day after your fast, you're open to choose from a variety of whole fresh fruits, simple salads, smoothies, and blended raw soups, as well as a variety of other healthy raw meal options. You can begin eating other fruits, too. Bananas, berries, mango, and pineapple are good options. Just be sure to avoid fats on this day, including oils, olives, and even avocados.

Start each morning with some whole fruit, a smoothie, or juice, and consume your largest meal midday. Then you can wrap up the day with a small, simple meal to ensure proper and complete digestion throughout the night.

On day 3, you can resume a relatively normal, healthy diet as long as you stay away from rich foods such as meat, dairy, and heavily processed foods. Start introducing fats back into your diet slowly. Your first meal of the day could include an avocado, some coconut, or olives if you like. Choose just one fat per meal on day 3, and only eat a small amount of it.

It's imperative to the success of your fast to follow through on these preparations for beginning and ending your juice fast rather than jumping right in or ending it with a veggie burger, a bowl of yogurt, or tofu scramble. Doing so would sabotage your efforts. There's no point to fasting unless you end it the right way, and for optimum long-term health, we recommend keeping a plant-based diet. An excellent book to help support this diet change is *The Complete Idiot's Guide to Low-Fat Vegan Cooking*, also written by Bo Rinaldi. This book provides the information and recipes you need to stay healthy, satisfied, and nutritionally balanced.

The Least You Need to Know

- Choosing an ideal environment is essential to your juice-fasting success, as is creating a support network.
- Making the perfect juice takes trial and error.
- You can juice fast even if you don't own a juicer.
- Eating simply before a fast helps improve your results.
- Breaking a fast with simple foods is absolutely imperative.

Short-Term Juice Fasting

Chapter 5

In This Chapter

- Introductory juice fasts
- Deciding which juice fast is best for you
- Eating before and after your juice fast
- Easy and effective short juice fasts

In previous chapters, we covered the multitude of benefits you'll gain from a juice fast of any length. In those chapters, we provided comprehensive information about weight loss and detoxification. In this chapter, we cover all the how's and when's for choosing the perfect introduction to juice fasting and including it in your ongoing health maintenance program.

If you're new to juice fasting, we recommend you begin with these shorter fasts before working your way up to longer ones. Bookmark and revisit this chapter often as you make progress toward longer juice fasts. They're the perfect way to make juice fasting a lifelong healthy habit. We hope this chapter inspires you to juice fast often and regularly to support your ever-increasing health.

Single-Day Juice Fasting

Single-day juice fasting is perfect for anyone for a variety of reasons. It's the most ideal way to understand the power of juice fasting. By committing to a 1-day juice fast, you'll see that you can fast without worrying about feeling hungry or low on energy. Sticking to a simple

1-day juice fast keeps you from getting in over your head with a larger commitment that could be hard to keep. After your first successful juice fast, you'll be more likely to try another and have continued success.

JUICY FACT

When you chew and digest solid food, your body has to work to extract the nutrients—the juice—from the cellular structure of the solids. By drinking juice, your body can skip that step. And that's why you'll find yourself with tons of energy while you juice fast. All the hard work has already been done for you so your body has more energy reserved for play.

A single-day juice fast is also easier to fit into your busy schedule. You can plan a single-day juice fast into your workweek and make your juices in the morning to bring along with you to the office. Or you could juice fast over a weekend. You could even plan a small retreat for yourself and turn your juice fast day into a health spa day. Get a massage, go for a short walk in the woods, sunbathe, or just do whatever makes you feel peaceful and rested. You can start 1-day juice fasts anytime you feel you need rejuvenation and want to give your body a break.

The "Whenever You Feel Like It" Fast

Having a plan for an "anytime" juice fast is essential if you decide on the fly that you feel like fasting. Maybe you want to wipe out an oncoming cold before you get sick. Or you may fast a couple days before a date so your skin is radiant and you feel more confident about your appearance. Perhaps you want to fast after a holiday, especially if you overindulged in heavy fare. A short fast is always beneficial for your health.

Optimally, the 2 days before your fast, you should eat more lightly and get your body ready for it, as detailed in Chapter 4. Also, don't forget those 2 days after your fast. You need to ease back into your "normal" eating style.

If you're in a pinch and you really just need a break from eating *now*, you could consume a liquid diet of fresh smoothies and/or raw vegan soups the day before your fast as well as a day or two after. This gives you an immediate break from eating solids, and your digestive system still gets some time to transition from a diet of solid foods to juices.

Use this quick "whenever you feel like it" fast to rest your digestive system and regain some natural vigor and energy without having to plan too far in advance:

Day 1:

> *Breakfast:* 16-ounce Berry Smoothie (Chapter 7)
>
> *Lunch:* Creamy Kale Soup (Chapter 7)
>
> *Snack:* Any 32-ounce juice from Chapter 9 or 10
>
> *Dinner:* 32-ounce Green Smoothie (Chapter 7)

Day 2:

> *Breakfast:* Any 32-ounce juice from Chapter 9
>
> *Lunch:* Any 32-ounce juice from Chapter 8, 11, or 12
>
> *Snack:* Any 32-ounce juice from Chapter 9
>
> *Dinner:* Any 32-ounce juice from Chapter 10

Day 3:

> *Breakfast:* Any 32-ounce juice from Chapter 9, 10, 11, or 12
>
> *Lunch:* 32-ounce Green Smoothie (Chapter 7)
>
> *Snack:* Any 32-ounce juice from any chapter
>
> *Dinner:* Raw Spinach Soup (Chapter 7)

Juice Fasting 1 Day a Week

An ideal way to lose weight at a steady, healthy pace while continuously improving your overall health is to commit to juice fasting 1 day every week. By doing so, you can make an ongoing commitment to constantly improving your health not only through juice fasting but also by following the meal plans that are integral to these protocols. This will help you improve your overall diet and your weight-loss goals.

TANTALIZING TIP

A 1-day juice fast done every week can actually do more for your health in the long run than if you just did one or two long fasts. You might be fasting for a small amount of time, but the frequency and regularity of your weekly juice fast has far-reaching healing effects.

This is a realistic and beneficial lifestyle change you can commit to for the rest of your life. Whatever your current diet might be like, whether it's the standard American diet, vegetarian, vegan, or raw vegan, you can easily shift your eating habits to include weekly juice fasting.

As your body begins to tune with the rhythm of your eating versus fasting days, you'll cleanse more effectively and lose weight more efficiently. Your body will start to anticipate your weekly juice fast cleanse as the day approaches and will make good use of this time. Just this minor change can bring unprecedented relief to digestive system disorders and other acute ailments. This new habit also can help curb tendencies to overeat throughout the rest of the week.

When you decide to incorporate weekly juice fasting into your ongoing health maintenance program, you should invest in a few inspiring cookbooks. We recommend Bo's other books, *The Complete Idiot's Guide to Eating Raw*, *The Complete Idiot's Guide to Low-Fat Vegan Cooking*, and *The Complete Idiot's Guide to Green Smoothies*. These books will give you ideas for meals and snacks that work well before and after your fasts.

Once you get into the routine of juice fasting, you can figure out which wholesome yet cleansing recipes—such as the recipes in Chapter 7—you like best. Then using our plan as a model, you can start to develop your own meal plans for your pre- and postfast days, letting your personal preferences be your guide. This helps keep your daily menu new and interesting while you continue your cleansing process. Just remember to keep your meals light before and after your weekly fast and refer to this section as a general template to guide your daily meal plans.

Here's a suggested meal plan for your 1-day-a-week juice-fasting protocol:

Day 1:

> *Breakfast:* 16-ounce Green Smoothie (Chapter 7)
>
> *Lunch:* Spinach Apple Soup and No Bean Raw Hummus (Chapter 7) served with vegetable sticks
>
> *Snack:* Any 32-ounce juice from Chapter 9
>
> *Dinner:* Avocado Kale Salad (Chapter 7)

Day 2:

> *Breakfast:* Raw Waldorf Salad (Chapter 7)
>
> *Lunch:* Creamy Kale Soup (Chapter 7)
>
> *Snack:* Any 32-ounce juice from Chapter 8 or 10
>
> *Dinner:* Green Smoothie (Chapter 7)

TANTALIZING TIP

We like the idea of breaking a juice fast with a green smoothie because it's basically a juice with fiber. It seems like a natural progression and a fairly intuitive way to break a fast. Other good break-fast foods are melons of all kinds, grapes, and other watery, cleansing fruits like cucumber, apple, mango, and pear. Feel free to use any of these to break your fast.

Day 3:

> *Breakfast:* Any 32-ounce juice from Chapter 9
>
> *Lunch:* Any 32-ounce juice from Chapter 8, 10, 11, or 12
>
> *Snack:* Any 32-ounce juice from Chapter 9
>
> *Dinner:* Any 32-ounce juice from Chapter 10

Day 4:

> *Breakfast:* 32-ounce Green Smoothie (Chapter 7)
>
> *Lunch:* 16-ounce Berry Smoothie (Chapter 7)
>
> *Snack:* Any 32-ounce juice from Chapter 10
>
> *Dinner:* Raw Waldorf Salad (Chapter 7)

Day 5:

> *Breakfast:* 32-ounce Green Smoothie or Berry Smoothie (Chapter 7)
>
> *Lunch:* Avocado Kale Salad (Chapter 7)
>
> *Snack:* Any 32-ounce juice from Chapter 9
>
> *Dinner:* Raw Nori Submarine Sandwich and Super Mixed Green Salad (Chapter 7)

The 3-Day Juice Fast

A 3-day juice fast is a bit more involved than a 1-day juice fast, but it's nearly as easy to follow and it's a great way to take your juice fasting to the next level. With a 3-day fast, you begin to deepen your cleansing and detoxification, which helps you drop more weight than on a 1-day cleanse.

This short fast is an optimal way to see significant results for a variety of health issues without it becoming too overwhelming. It only takes about 3 days for your body to flush out toxins circulating in your lymph and circulatory systems. By day 2 of your juice fast, you'll begin to notice a smoother, clearer complexion. You'll also find improved elasticity and better tone for the skin over your entire body!

A 3-day juice fast is long enough to get great benefits, but isn't so long that you'll experience deep detoxification, which can bring on headaches or flulike symptoms. If you feel confident that you can get through a 3-day juice fast with no problem, feel free to use our Glowing Skin Juice Fast, later in this chapter, as the perfect introductory cleanse to your juice-fasting journey.

Getting Instant Results

A 3-day juice fast can be a wonderful treat for your body. With all likelihood, you'll have so much energy you won't even miss eating solid food. Instead, your body will feel light and you'll be greatly invigorated. You'll feel like you're glowing from the inside out, and don't be surprised if others comment on how radiant you look!

Within just a few days, you'll be able to see just how powerful juice fasting is for encouraging weight loss and improving any type of skin condition. You might not clear up an entire case of psoriasis with a 3-day fast, but you'll start to see immediate relief and regeneration enough to inspire you to try a longer fast in the future. No other method of cleansing provides such profound results so quickly as a juice fast.

PULPY PITFALL

Conditions like psoriasis are, at their root, caused by an overgrowth of candida. This fungus normally lives harmoniously in the body until the body becomes acidic, which stimulates candida growth. Sugar feeds candida, so if you have inflammatory skin conditions and are searching for relief, stay away from juices high in sugar. Instead, drink juice recipes that include more cucumber or celery and other watery or green vegetables.

This 3-day juice fast is no miracle cure, but you're sure to notice almost immediate differences in the way you look and feel. It's an instant boost to your confidence and your health alike, and you'll be feeling younger and spryer than you can remember. There's no reason to delay your next juice fast!

The Glowing Skin Juice Fast

This is truly a gem of a program. We all want to feel great and look youthful. Juice fasting can help achieve this by smoothing over wrinkles, clearing up acne, and toning your skin. In just 3 days, you'll notice vast improvement in chronic or acute skin conditions such as eczema, psoriasis, or even a persistent case of athlete's foot.

If you partake in this juice fast regularly, you'll notice your skin will take on a rosy complexion. This is because the vitamins, minerals, and phytonutrients in your fresh juices will flood your system with nutrition and impart a healthy glow all over your body. As an added benefit, when you get some sun exposure, you'll be far more resistant to sunburn. All those micronutrients and omega fatty acids in your juices are nature's version of sunscreen. They work far better than anything you can buy in a bottle!

This is an extremely effective fast to do any time you want to look your best. It's a perfect way to slim down as you prepare for the summer months. You can perform this juice fast once a month, every other month, or at any other interval that feels comfortable to you.

Here's your menu:

Day 1:

> *Breakfast:* 2 or 3 cups fresh fruit
>
> *Lunch:* Creamy Kale Soup (Chapter 7)
>
> *Snack:* Any 32-ounce juice from Chapter 10 or 11
>
> *Dinner:* Green Smoothie (Chapter 7)

Days 2 through 4:

> *Breakfast:* Any 32-ounce juice containing pineapple, melon, turmeric, ginger, wheatgrass, or *noni*

DEFINITION

Noni is a tropical fruit native to Hawaii and the Polynesian islands. It resembles a large smooth, white mulberry and has a taste and smell you'll never forget. The flavor is reminiscent of apple cider vinegar and jackfruit with onionlike tones and a slightly salty aftertaste. Noni has been used traditionally by the native Polynesians to heal flesh wounds and any type of digestive disorder.

> *Lunch:* 32 ounces of Carrot Apple Lemon Juice, Cucumber Apple Celery Cilantro Juice, Carrot Parsley Cabbage Juice, or Carrot Parsley Beet Juice (Chapter 9)

Snack: Any 32-ounce juice from Chapter 8, 10, 11, or 12

Dinner: Any 32-ounce juice from Chapter 9 or 10

Day 5:

Breakfast: Any 32-ounce juice from Chapter 10

Lunch: ½ small melon of your choice, blended

Snack: Any 32-ounce juice from Chapter 9 or 10

Dinner: 32-ounce Green Smoothie (Chapter 7)

Day 6:

Breakfast: 32-ounce Green Smoothie (Chapter 7)

Lunch: 16-ounce Berry Smoothie (Chapter 7)

Snack: Fresh fruit and/or any 32-ounce juice from Chapter 10

Dinner: Creamy Kale Soup (Chapter 7)

The Once-a-Month Rejuvenation Fast

We all need to spend some time now and then taking care of our health. We become so busy in our daily lives that we often neglect to give our bodies the tender love and care we deserve. A juice fast is a great way to make up for what we neglect on a daily basis. Incorporating this 3-day juice fast, combined with a 6-day raw vegan diet, gives your digestive system a rest, providing your body with some needed rejuvenation every month. We can all use that!

TANTALIZING TIP

Raw foods contain living enzymes that help the food digest itself rather than deplete your finite enzymes stores. Enzymes also help cleanse your body of plaque and toxins, so eating raw foods for several days before your juice fast gives you a head start on your cleansing and detoxification process. This simple step is essential for getting the most benefit from your juice fast.

For this particular fast, we recommend consuming only raw vegan foods for several days leading up to your 3-day fast. This gives your body more time to begin preparing for your fast and greatly enhances the benefits of your juice fast. This is only necessary if you plan to incorporate this particular juice fast as part of your regular routine.

Here's your menu:

Day 1:

> *Breakfast:* 16-ounce Berry Smoothie (Chapter 7)
>
> *Lunch:* Avocado Boats (Chapter 7) and 16 ounces of any juice from Chapter 10
>
> *Snack:* No Bean Raw Hummus (Chapter 7) served with vegetable sticks
>
> *Dinner:* Avocado Kale Salad (Chapter 7)

Day 2:

> *Breakfast:* 32-ounce Green Smoothie (Chapter 7)
>
> *Lunch:* Raw Submarine Sandwich (Chapter 7)
>
> *Snack:* Any 32-ounce juice from Chapter 9
>
> *Dinner:* Mixed Green Salad (Chapter 7)

Day 3:

> *Breakfast:* Any 32-ounce juice from Chapter 9
>
> *Lunch:* 32-ounce Green Smoothie (Chapter 7)
>
> *Snack:* Any 32-ounce juice from Chapter 8, 10, 11, or 12
>
> *Dinner:* 32-ounce Green Smoothie (Chapter 7)

Days 4 through 6:

> *Breakfast:* Any 32-ounce juice from Chapter 9
>
> *Lunch:* Any 32-ounce juice from Chapter 10
>
> *Snack:* Any 32-ounce juice from Chapter 9
>
> *Dinner:* Any 32-ounce juice from Chapter 8, 10, 11, or 12

Day 7:

>*Breakfast:* 16-ounce Green Smoothie (Chapter 7)
>
>*Lunch:* 16-ounce Berry Smoothie (Chapter 7)
>
>*Snack:* Any 32-ounce juice from Chapter 8, 10, 11, or 12
>
>*Dinner:* 2 or 3 cups fresh fruit

>**JUICY FACT**
>
>Nearly all fruits and vegetables are alkalizing. Because most diseases thrive in an acidic environment, alkalizing your body with fresh juices is one of the most important things you can do to prevent and reverse disease.

Day 8:

>*Breakfast:* 32-ounce Green Smoothie or Berry Smoothie (Chapter 7)
>
>*Lunch:* Creamy Kale Salad (Chapter 7)
>
>*Snack:* Any 32-ounce juice from Chapter 9
>
>*Dinner:* Super Mixed Green Salad (Chapter 7)

Day 9:

>*Breakfast:* 32-ounce Green Smoothie or Berry Smoothie (Chapter 7)
>
>*Lunch:* Spinach Apple Soup (Chapter 7)
>
>*Snack:* Any 32-ounce juice from Chapter 9
>
>*Dinner:* Raw Nori Submarine Sandwich and Avocado Boats (Chapter 7)

The 7-Day Juice Fast

We recommend a 7-day juice fast for ongoing health maintenance and to keep your body at its fittest. It's also the perfect way to give your body a chance to go deeper with your cleansing, especially if you can't commit to weekly single-day juice fasts. You can complete this longer fast less frequently and receive very similar benefits. You may find that you have a better response to the cleansing benefits of this longer fast and in theory, the longer you cleanse, the more deeply you clean out your system. Juice fasting for an entire week brings about more significant changes than you might experience from shorter fasts. Also, you can expect to lose some serious weight in a short time and keep those extra pounds at bay.

When cleansing at such a deep level, many people experience some uncomfortable detox reactions often referred to as a healing crisis. It's not uncommon for your body to feel achy, to experience headaches, or to have an overall feeling of discomfort as your body eliminates deeper toxins.

If you start experiencing these symptoms and you want some relief, replace your fruit juices and green juices from Chapters 8, 10, 11, and 12 with more of the grounding, nutrient-dense juices in Chapter 9, which will help slow down your detox process to a more comfortable pace. Also, try enemas and colonics to help cleanse your body faster. When you're cleansing on such a deep level, the toxins aren't able to leave your body fast enough and the flulike symptoms result. If you speed up the process with an enema or colonic, you'll feel better immediately as the toxins pour from your body faster.

As far as juice fasts go, the 7-day fast is excellent for the more seasoned fasters, although you also could use our Vibrant Body Juice Fast as your first juice fast. You'll get amazing results as long as you stay committed through the end. For those experiencing a serious health issue, you may want to ask your health professional if you can perform a 7-day juice fast to start your recovery process right away. This juice fast is the perfect protocol for longevity and perfect health.

Fasting 1 Week a Month

Although it might sound overwhelming right now, before you've started your first juice fast, believe us when we tell you regular week-long juice fasts every month yield some serious long-term health benefits. Giving your body the chance to remove the toxins stored in your tissues adds years to your life and protects you from age-related, auto-immune, and degenerative diseases, including cancer. Forget about your family's medical history, and juice-fast your way to a thriving, healthy, perfect body.

Juice fasting for an entire week every month is the perfect way to maintain the benefits you get from longer fasts. With monthly fasts, you continue your cleansing without having the need to complete longer cleanse programs. Maintaining a commitment to a monthly weeklong fast keeps you from sliding back into old habits and prevents your body from accumulating toxins in the future.

PULPY PITFALL

Juice fasting is a wonderful way to periodically cleanse your body and can be an ideal way to start implementing healthy changes in your diet. But beware of jumping into a fast without much of a plan on how to maintain your health afterward. Coming off your juice fast and returning to poor eating habits will just make you gain back any lost weight.

Juice fast for a week every month, and soon, what seems like a fast will transform into a pleasant and healthy habit. Of course, you shouldn't feel restricted to fasting for just 1 week during the month. You can always choose to fast 1 week on and 1 week off until you intuitively feel it's time to cut it back to once a month again.

The Vibrant Body Juice Fast

This 7-day fasting program was designed as a short yet effective health overhaul. When you start experiencing chronic symptoms such as psoriasis, insomnia, depression, or other mysterious and unexplainable illnesses, use this fast to restore yourself to vibrant health.

Here's your menu:

Day 1:

> *Breakfast:* 16-ounce Berry Smoothie (Chapter 7)
>
> *Lunch:* Raw Nori Submarine Sandwich (Chapter 7)
>
> *Snack:* 16 ounces of any juice from Chapter 9 and No Bean Raw Hummus (Chapter 7) served with vegetable sticks
>
> *Dinner:* Avocado Boats and Raw Creamy Pea Soup (Chapter 7)

Day 2:

> *Breakfast:* Raw Waldorf Salad (Chapter 7)
>
> *Lunch:* Creamy Kale Soup (Chapter 7)
>
> *Snack:* Any 32-ounce juice from Chapter 9 or 10 or a 16-ounce Berry Smoothie (Chapter 7)
>
> *Dinner:* 16-ounce Green Smoothie (Chapter 7)

Days 3 through 9:

> *Breakfast:* Any 32-ounce juice from Chapter 8 containing pineapple, grapefruit, or kiwi
>
> *Lunch:* Any 32-ounce juice from Chapter 10
>
> *Snack:* Any 32-ounce juice from Chapter 9
>
> *Dinner:* Any 32-ounce juice from Chapter 10, 11, or 12

Day 10:

> *Breakfast:* ½ small melon of choice, blended
>
> *Lunch:* 16 ounces of any juice from Chapter 10
>
> *Snack:* ½ small melon of choice, blended
>
> *Dinner:* 16-ounce Green Smoothie (Chapter 7)

Day 11:

> *Breakfast:* ½ small melon of choice
>
> *Lunch:* Any 32-ounce juice from any chapter
>
> *Snack:* 16-ounce Berry Smoothie (Chapter 7)
>
> *Dinner:* 32-ounce Green Smoothie (Chapter 7)

TANTALIZING TIP

Melons are one of the most easily digested foods on the planet. Because they take no effort to digest, melons place no stress on your digestive system and very gently break your fast.

No matter the reason or the season, you can jumpstart your health and healing *now* with one of these juice fasts. Try one, or try them all. Use them as stepping-stones toward longer fasts, or familiarize yourself with one or two and stick with them. If your goal is to live with vitality coursing through your body and overwhelming joy in your heart, you've come to the right place.

The Least You Need to Know

- Short-term juice fasts are the best way to learn how to juice fast successively.
- You can do an intermittent juice fast any time you feel you need to cleanse *now*.
- Regular short juice fasts are very effective in the long term.
- Making juice fasting a part of your healthy lifestyle is the best way to experience lasting health.

Long-Term Juice *Feasting*

In This Chapter

- Feasting on fresh juice
- Taking your juice fast to the next level
- Meal plans for before and after your juice fast
- Plans for long-term juice fasting

When you decide to embark on a long-term juice fast lasting more than a week or two, you should do so with care but still with confidence. There's no harm in starting small, so give yourself time to work up to the juice fasts in this chapter.

We've found that long-term juice fasting can be the most effective way to combat any health disorders. This is particularly true if you make a commitment to one or two longer juice fasts every year with some intermittent shorter fasts in between.

A Sample Juice-Fasting Holiday

During these longer cleanses, it's important to allow yourself time to rest and take in the benefits of your juice fast. It's also important to manage your time wisely to avoid stress and to schedule in some extra home therapies while cleansing to stimulate your blood flow and support your detox. We've provided a sample of what our days look like while on a juice-fasting holiday.

Upon waking: You can take an enema, followed by massaging your skin with a dry brush from your extremities toward your heart. Wrap it up with a shower alternating between hot and cold water. To do this, make your shower temperature warm/hot as usual. After a few minutes, turn down the warm/hot and stand in cold water for as long as you can tolerate. Repeat this four or five times during your shower. Showering this way during your cleanse improves your circulation, which is essential in helping push out accumulated waste from your body faster. Other benefits include strengthened immunity, improved skin and hair, alleviation from depression, and increased fertility.

8 A.M.: Drink a cup of warm (not hot) herbal tea. We recommend chamomile, peppermint, smooth move, rose hips, or any other herbs you plan on using during your cleanse.

10 A.M.: Drink 32 ounces freshly pressed green/vegetable juice.

11 A.M.: Engage in mild exercise such as walking, yoga, light weight-lifting, rebounding, etc., until about 1 P.M. followed by sunbathing, if weather permits.

1 P.M.: Drink 32 ounces freshly pressed fruit juice straight, or diluted 50/50 with filtered water.

1:30 P.M.: We highly recommend you use this time for creative productivity and self-expression like reading a good book, making art or music, meditating, or even taking a nap if that's what your body tells you it needs.

4 P.M.: Drink 32 ounces freshly pressed green juice.

4:30 P.M.: Take an aromatherapy bath, do some light exercise, get a massage, etc.

6 P.M.: Drink 32 ounces freshly pressed green/vegetable juice.

Evening: Rest.

TANTALIZING TIP

On any juice fast you choose, drink filtered water whenever you're thirsty. You can dilute fruit juices with filtered water to lower the sugar content, but never dilute vegetable or green juices. You want all those precious nutrients.

The 28-Day Juice Fast

A 28-day juice fast is a month-long miracle program for health and healing. Countless numbers of people have lost unwanted weight and healed a variety of health issues in this period of time. Going all out on a 28-day juice fast gives your body an extended chance for deep cleansing, thereby pulling out stagnant toxic material and reviving your healthy tissues.

Everyone's body has different factors that will determine exactly how fast they detox and how quickly they melt off the pounds, but over a month of juice fasting, your health will be better than you can ever remember. It's not uncommon for a long fast like this to eradicate diseases of all kinds. Of course, if you're trying to heal yourself of any disease, you should talk to your health-care provider about your intentions first and have regular checkups with him or her through-out your cleanse.

Don't be afraid to get a second opinion if your doctor isn't onboard with your juice fasting. Although juice fasting is a safe method of healing for *most* people, many medical professionals have biased opinions toward natural healing. If your physician doesn't support your efforts, plenty of others are familiar with juice fasting and can help advise you. Just give your regular doctor a copy of this book so he can learn more about juice fasting and find someone else who is more qualified to advise you.

Working Up to a 28-Day Juice Fast

If you've never juice fasted before, contemplating a 28-day juice fast may seem a bit daunting. Such a reaction is perfectly normal, but remember, juice fasting is a perfectly safe and natural method for healing. The idea of experiencing flulike "detox reactions" and craving solid foods may seem like big hurdles to conquer, but the whole process is much easier and more pleasant than you can imagine.

It's not a bad idea to work your way up to a longer fast like this, and it's actually wise to try a series of shorter fasts before going all out on a 28-day juice fast.

You could approach this longer type of fast by doing a series of shorter fasts over a relatively short period of time. For example, you could start with a 1-day fast and then try a 3-day fast a week later. If all goes well, over the following week or two, you could go on a 7-day juice fast and then start your 28-day fast within the next month.

Another option is to space out your short fasts over a longer period of time so your body becomes accustomed to the feeling of fasting. Let's say you've already done a few short fasts and now you're working up to a week-long juice fast. You could do one week-long juice fast every month for 6 months and then try a 28-day fast.

Still, it may take you years of shorter fasts to get comfortable enough to do a long fast, and that's perfectly okay. Use your intuition when choosing a fast, and only commit to what you know you can stick with until you gain confidence and familiarity with the juice-fasting process.

The "Fountain of Youth" Fast

This is truly the grandmaster of juice fasts, so get ready to set back the clock and unleash more boundless energy than you ever knew was inside you!

As we discussed earlier in this chapter, you might want to prepare for this cleanse by completing several shorter juice fasts. Be sure you're mentally prepared to complete this 28-day fast. Performing shorter cleanses makes you more likely to stick with this longer fast and also deepens your cleanse, resulting in more healing, rejuvenation, and restored vigor.

You can do this fast several times a year for the best results. You may want to try it twice in a year or possibly bump it up to three or four times. This is going to be particularly effective for those working on healing chronic illness. If you're following a simple raw or predominantly raw vegan diet between several of these juice fasts, you'll be in amazing health in no time.

Here's your menu:

Day 1:

> *Breakfast:* 2 cups fresh fruit
>
> *Lunch:* Raw Nori Submarine Sandwich (Chapter 7)
>
> *Snack:* 16 ounces of any juice from Chapter 9
>
> *Dinner:* Avocado Boats and Super Mixed Green Salad (Chapter 7)

Day 2:

> *Breakfast:* Berry Smoothie (Chapter 7)
>
> *Lunch:* 16 ounces of any juice from Chapter 8, 9, or 10 and Raw Waldorf Salad (Chapter 7)
>
> *Snack:* 16 ounces of any juice from Chapter 9
>
> *Dinner:* Creamy Kale Soup (Chapter 7)

Day 3:

> *Breakfast:* Any 32-ounce juice from Chapter 10
>
> *Lunch:* 32-ounce Berry Smoothie (Chapter 7)
>
> *Snack:* 16 ounces of any juice from Chapter 9
>
> *Dinner:* 32-ounce Green Smoothie (Chapter 7)

Days 4 through 31:

> *Breakfast:* Any 32-ounce juice from Chapter 9
>
> *Lunch:* Any 32-ounce juice from Chapter 8, 10, 11, or 12
>
> *Snack:* Any 32-ounce juice from Chapter 9
>
> *Dinner:* Any 32-ounce juice from Chapter 10, 11, or 12

PULPY PITFALL

For longer juice fasts like a 28-day fast, we recommend you drink at least two vegetable-based juices a day from Chapter 9 to be sure you're flooding your body with green nutrients, which in turn will keep you mentally focused and your energy high. Fruit juices are highly cleansing and can exacerbate detox symptoms.

Day 32:

Breakfast: ½ small melon of choice, blended

Lunch: Any 32-ounce juice from Chapter 10

Snack: ½ small melon of choice, blended

Dinner: 32-ounce Green Smoothie (Chapter 7)

Day 33:

Breakfast: 32-ounce Green Smoothie (Chapter 7)

Lunch: 2 or 3 cups of any fresh fruit

Snack: Any 32-ounce juice from any chapter

Dinner: Berry Smoothie (Chapter 7)

Day 34:

Breakfast: 32-ounce Green Smoothie (Chapter 7)

Lunch: Spinach Apple Soup (Chapter 7)

Snack: Raw Waldorf Salad (Chapter 7)

Dinner: Avocado Kale Salad (Chapter 7)

Long-Term Juice Feasting

As you learn more about juice fasting, don't be surprised to hear about very long juice fasts—up to 100 days and even longer in some cases! These go beyond mere juice fasts and are more like juice *feasts*. On these longer programs, you wash your body clean and allow it a fresh start at life without the burden of toxins and sluggish digestion.

When you've become more experienced with juice fasting, you can try juice feasting if you like. Every juice recipe in this book can be included in a juice feast.

TANTALIZING TIP

If you concentrate on what you're giving up and what you miss about your old diet and lifestyle while you juice fast, you'll certainly feel like you're missing out and you might not have the motivation to keep going with your fast. Instead, change your mind-set and focus on your reasons for beginning the fast. Think about what you're getting out of it instead. The success stories in Appendix C will motivate you when you learn how many people overcame unbelievable circumstances simply through juice fasting. With a positive outlook, you can do anything!

When embarking on a juice fast lasting more than a month, you may want to enlist the help of a trusted and supportive medical professional. Most people can partake in long-term juice fasting without adverse reactions, but those with preexisting medical conditions should be monitored throughout the fast. Even if you're generally healthy, it's a good idea to have someone look after your well-being during your long-term juice feast. In Appendix B, we share some websites and professionals who can help guide you during your extended juice feast.

The Radical Fast

As the name suggests, this fast might seem a bit radical, but we assure you it's just as safe and even more effective for healing than the fasts we've given you up to this point. This fast lasts 40 days and is book-ended by 3 days of transition diet before and after the fast.

This fast is the go-to cure-it-all fast and is a good option for those who have been assigned to a lifetime of medication for chronic illnesses. Just one or two of these fasts can do wonders for your health. This fast can alleviate many autoimmune diseases like lupus and even may be helpful for Lyme disease and a host of "incurable" viruses like those that cause hepatitis.

To better prepare your body for such a long fast, we recommend you eliminate all dairy and meat from your diet 1 month prior to beginning the fast. You should also cut out wheat and other products containing gluten and also remove any refined sugar from your diet at least 2 weeks before you begin. Try to maintain a diet as close to a high-raw vegan diet as you can for the remaining 2 weeks. This helps lessen the detox symptoms you'll experience during your cleanse.

Here's your menu:

Day 1:

> *Breakfast:* 16-ounce Berry Smoothie (Chapter 7)
>
> *Lunch:* Raw Nori Submarine Sandwich (Chapter 7)
>
> *Snack:* 16 ounces of any juice from Chapter 9
>
> *Dinner:* Avocado Boats and Super Mixed Green Salad (Chapter 7)

Day 2:

> *Breakfast:* 2 cups fresh fruit
>
> *Lunch:* 16 ounces of any juice from Chapter 8, 11, or 12 and Super Mixed Green Salad (Chapter 7)
>
> *Snack:* 16 ounces of any juice from Chapter 9 or 2 cups fresh fruit
>
> *Dinner:* Creamy Kale Soup (Chapter 7)

Day 3:

> *Breakfast:* Any 32-ounce juice from Chapter 10
>
> *Lunch:* 2 or 3 cups fresh fruit
>
> *Snack:* 16 ounces of any juice from Chapter 9
>
> *Dinner:* 32-ounce Green Smoothie (Chapter 7)

JUICY FACT

Ending your transition diet with a green smoothie is the perfect way to launch into your healing juice fast. The fruit and fiber give your colon an effective cleansing and prepare it for your upcoming deep detox.

Days 4 through 22:

Early morning: 8 ounces herbal tea (see recommended herbs in Chapter 3) with 1 tablespoon bentonite or zeolite plus 2 teaspoons *psyllium husk;* stir and drink before psyllium gels

Breakfast: Any 32-ounce juice from Chapter 9

Lunch: Any 32-ounce juice from Chapter 8, 10, 11, or 12

Snack: Any 32-ounce juice from Chapter 9

Dinner: Any 32-ounce juice from Chapter 10

DEFINITION

Psyllium husk are the casings of small seeds that gel, similar to the way flax and chia gel. It's great for cleansing the blood and intestines.

Days 23 through 29:

Early morning: 8 ounces herbal tea with 1 tablespoon bentonite or zeolite stirred in

Breakfast: Any 32-ounce juice from Chapter 10 (stir in 3 tablespoons chia seeds and allow to soak for 10 minutes)

Lunch: Any 32-ounce juice from Chapter 9 (stir in 3 tablespoons chia seeds and allow to soak for 10 minutes)

Snack: Any 32-ounce juice from Chapter 8, 10, 11, or 12 (stir in 3 tablespoons chia seeds and allow to soak for 10 minutes)

Dinner: Any 32-ounce juice from Chapter 10

Days 30 through 43:

Early morning: 8 ounces herbal tea with 1 tablespoon bentonite or zeolite plus 2 teaspoons psyllium husk; stir and drink before psyllium gels

Breakfast: Any 32-ounce juice from Chapter 9

Lunch: Any 32-ounce juice from Chapter 8, 10, 11, or 12

Snack: Any 32-ounce juice from Chapter 9

Dinner: Any 32-ounce juice from Chapter 10

Day 44:

Breakfast: 1 or 2 small pieces of fruit such as ½ small melon or 2 small peaches, blended

Lunch: Any 32-ounce juice from Chapter 9, 10, or 11

Snack: 32-ounce Green Smoothie (Chapter 7)

Dinner: 2 cups fresh fruit (Chapter 7)

Day 45:

Breakfast: As much fresh fruit as you like

Lunch: Super Mixed Green Salad (Chapter 7)

Snack: As much fresh fruit as you like or 16 ounces any juice from any chapter

Dinner: 16-ounce Green Smoothie (Chapter 7)

Day 46:

Breakfast: 16-ounce Berry Smoothie (Chapter 7)

Lunch: Creamy Kale Soup (Chapter 7)

Snack: Any 32-ounce juice from any chapter

Dinner: Avocado Kale Salad (Chapter 7)

The Ultra-Radical Fast

As with the previous fasting protocol, this is not a fast to be taken lightly. We recommend this fast as a curative program for those with chronic illness. It can also be used as a last-resort treatment for those whom Western medicine can no longer help. Countless individuals with stage 4 cancer and other terminal illnesses have made a full recovery with a long-term fast like this.

This is a 90-day juice-fasting protocol. If you ever feel like you need to lessen the detox effects of your fast but still want to keep up your healing process, add 2 tablespoons chia seeds to your fresh juice and allow it to sit until it gels. You could also try blending your juice ingredients and drinking them with the fiber included for a day or two at a time. This gives you the sensation of being fuller longer and won't stop your cleanse but will still help manage detox symptoms. If you do blend your juice ingredients for a few days, choose recipes that don't contain too much carrot, beet, or apple because the resulting texture might not be particularly appetizing. Instead, choose juices with melon, pear, citrus, and other softer ingredients.

Try to expose as much of your skin to the fresh air and sunshine as often as you can. Get regular massages at least once a week, and do a few colonics to ensure you're getting the most out of your cleanse. These complementary treatments will help your body safely remove toxins more quickly and effectively.

Here's your menu:

Day 1:

> *Breakfast:* 16-ounce Berry Smoothie (Chapter 7)
>
> *Lunch:* Raw Nori Submarine Sandwich (Chapter 7)
>
> *Snack:* 16 ounces of any juice from Chapter 9
>
> *Dinner:* Avocado Boats and Super Mixed Green Salad (Chapter 7)

Day 2:

> *Breakfast:* 2 cups fresh fruit
>
> *Lunch:* 16 ounces of any juice from Chapter 8, 11, or 12 and Super Mixed Green Salad (Chapter 7)
>
> *Snack:* 16 ounces of any juice from Chapter 9 or 2 cups fresh fruit
>
> *Dinner:* Creamy Kale Soup (Chapter 7)

PULPY PITFALL

Don't go into a long-term juice feast with fear that you can't complete it. Instead, tackle smaller goals and work up to longer fasts later. You can start by committing to a 28-day fast and then if you feel like you can keep going, extend it to a 40-day or even a 90-day juice fast. Just don't let doubt creep in and sabotage your efforts.

Day 3:

Breakfast: Any 32-ounce juice from Chapter 10

Lunch: 2 or 3 cups fresh fruit

Snack: 16 ounces of any juice from Chapter 9

Dinner: 32-ounce Green Smoothie (Chapter 7)

Days 4 through 94:

Early morning: 8 ounces herbal tea with 1 tablespoon bentonite or zeolite plus 2 teaspoons psyllium husk; stir and drink before psyllium gels

Breakfast: Any 32-ounce juice from Chapter 9

Lunch: Any 32-ounce juice from Chapter 8, 10, 11, or 12

Snack: Any 32-ounce juice from Chapter 9

Dinner: Any 32-ounce juice from Chapter 10, 11, or 12

Before bed: 8 ounces herbal tea with 1 tablespoon bentonite or zeolite plus 2 teaspoons psyllium husk; stir and drink before psyllium gels

Day 95:

Breakfast: 1 or 2 small pieces of fruit such as ½ small melon, 1 large pear, 2 small peaches, or a small bunch of grapes, blended

Lunch: Any 32-ounce juice from Chapter 10

Snack: 32-ounce Green Smoothie (Chapter 7)

Dinner: 2 cups fresh fruit (Chapter 7)

Day 96:

Breakfast: As much fresh fruit as you like

Lunch: 16-ounce Green Smoothie (Chapter 7)

Snack: About 2 cups fresh fruit or 16 ounces of any juice from any chapter

Dinner: Super Mixed Green Salad (Chapter 7)

Day 97:

> *Breakfast:* As much fresh fruit as you like
>
> *Lunch:* 16-ounce Berry Smoothie (Chapter 7)
>
> *Snack:* Any 32-ounce juice from any chapter
>
> *Dinner:* Creamy Kale Soup (Chapter 7)

It's our sincere hope that you find the inspiration you need to carry you through any health challenge within the pages of this book. These extended juice fasts will provide the guidance you need to complete your own healing juice fast. Long-term juice fasts will help you find strength you never knew you had and inspire you to live life with joy and integrity. They are truly life-changing.

The Least You Need to Know

- You can feel full and satisfied for months on a juice fast.
- Long-term juice fasting is very effective at healing your body.
- Long-term juice fasts are ideally done more than once a year.
- You can safely juice fast for as long as 90 days and beyond!

Terrific Transitional Recipes

In This Chapter

- Raw food recipes for transition days
- Sensational smoothies
- Nourishing soups, salads, and sandwiches
- Simple, healthy, and filling dishes

We felt it was important to offer you a few recipes to use in your transition diet between your normal eating habits and your juice-fasting days. These recipes prepare your body for juice fasting by encouraging your colon to remove waste and by helping your body adjust to eating lighter before beginning the juice fast. We hope you enjoy them as much as we do!

Feel free to use any of these recipes during your transition diet or replace them with similar items as you become more familiar with juice fasting.

Green Smoothie

Green smoothies are nourishing and taste great! This spinach, pineapple, and banana version can serve as a filling meal, lunch, or dinner. It has a wonderful sweet and tart yet mild flavor.

Yield:	Prep time:	Serving size:
about 4 cups	10 minutes	about 2 cups

Each serving has:		
232 calories	59 g carbohydrates	1 g fat
8 g fiber	4 g protein	117% vitamin A
225% vitamin C	10% calcium	27% magnesium
14% iron	29% potassium	

4 cups fresh spinach leaves	2 medium-large bananas, peeled
½ large pineapple, peeled, cored, and chopped (2 cups)	1½ cups filtered water

1. In a high-speed blender, combine spinach, pineapple, bananas, and water.

2. Blend until completely smooth.

JUICY FACT

The benefits of green smoothies have been well documented by raw food pioneer Dr. Ann Wigmore. In recent years, raw food educator Victoria Boutenko has performed studies and written books on the healing and detoxifying value of these mixtures. Also check out Bo's book *The Complete Idiot's Guide to Green Smoothies.*

Berry Smoothie

This vanilla-scented, sweet, slightly tart, and creamy smoothie can serve as a meal replacement or as a snack. The taste is dreamy, like a lost summer day at the beach.

Yield:	Prep time:	Serving size:
4 cups	15 minutes	2 cups

Each serving has:		
617 calories	99 g carbohydrates	25 g fat
12 g fiber	13 g protein	4% vitamin A
95% vitamin C	9% calcium	55% magnesium
28% iron	31% potassium	

2 cups fresh or frozen blueberries	6 medjool dates, pitted (about ½ cup)
1 cup fresh or frozen strawberries	1 vanilla bean, or 1 tsp. vanilla extract
½ cup raw cashews	1 cup filtered water

1. In a high-speed blender, combine blueberries, strawberries, cashews, medjool dates, vanilla bean, and water.

2. Blend until completely smooth.

TANTALIZING TIP

This delicious smoothie will keep for up to 2 days in the refrigerator, so prepare extra if you like. If you'd like to try a thicker, puddinglike version, add 3 tablespoons chia seeds to the blender.

Raw Creamy Corn Soup

This creamy and sweet soup is satisfying and silky. It's bursting with savory herbs and tons of flavor. You won't even realize this is a raw dish—it's that savory!

Yield:	Prep time:	Serving size:
about 4 cups	20 minutes	about 2 cups

Each serving has:		
323 calories	35 g carbohydrates	18 g fat
7 g fiber	13 g protein	117% vitamin A
59% vitamin C	4% calcium	35% magnesium
17% iron	17% potassium	

1¼ cups fresh or frozen corn kernels

¼ cup raw cashews

1 medium carrot, chopped

½ small red bell pepper, stem and seeds removed (¼ cup)

2 tsp. cold-pressed extra-virgin olive oil

2 cups filtered water

2 TB. nutritional yeast flakes

1 tsp. ground cumin

1 TB. red onion

1 small clove garlic

1 tsp. psyllium husks

½ tsp. Himalayan or Celtic sea salt

1 TB. fresh parsley, minced

Pinch freshly ground black pepper

1. In a high-speed blender, combine 1 cup corn kernels, cashews, carrot, red bell pepper, extra-virgin olive oil, water, nutritional yeast flakes, cumin, red onion, garlic, psyllium husks, and Himalayan sea salt.

2. Blend until a creamy consistency is reached and soup is slightly warm.

3. Add remaining ¼ cup corn kernels, parsley, and black pepper.

4. Serve immediately.

Raw Spinach Soup

This raw soup is creamy, it's zesty, and it has a bit of a pungent kick.
You'll savor every spoonful—and come back for more!

Yield:	Prep time:	Serving size:
about 3 cups	15 minutes	1½ cups

Each serving has:		
221 calories	14 g carbohydrates	18 g fat
7 g fiber	4 g protein	74% vitamin A
60% vitamin C	6% calcium	17% magnesium
11% iron	25% potassium	

2 cups fresh spinach leaves	¼ cup filtered water
1 large tomato, sliced	2 TB. coconut aminos
½ medium cucumber, peeled	½ tsp. Himalayan or Celtic sea salt
1 small avocado, pitted and peeled	1 TB. fresh lemon juice
1 small clove garlic	1 TB. cold-pressed extra-virgin olive oil
	Dash cayenne

1. In a high-speed blender, combine spinach, tomato, cucumber, avocado, garlic, water, coconut aminos, Himalayan sea salt, lemon juice, extra-virgin olive oil, and cayenne.

2. Blend until completely smooth.

JUICY FACT

Spinach is native to central and southwestern Asia. Its mild flavor makes it a favorite in anything from salads and soups to smoothies. It also happens to be packed with more protein per weight than beef or other meats and boasts a far greater array of alkalizing nutrients and healing properties.

Creamy Kale Soup

Tart lemon and creamy avocado combine beautifully with slightly pungent onion to create this exciting and flavorful green soup. You won't even realize how much nutritious green power your body is getting, but you'll feel it when you're done!

Yield:	Prep time:	Serving size:
about 2½ cups	15 minutes	2½ cups

Each serving has:		
893 calories	63 g carbohydrates	64 g fat
28 g fiber	39 g protein	827% vitamin A
565% vitamin C	63% calcium	100% magnesium
52% iron	68% potassium	

2 cups fresh almond milk	¼ small red onion, sliced (⅛ cup)
1 TB. fresh lemon juice	
½ medium avocado, pitted and peeled	2 TB. nutritional yeast flakes
4 medium kale leaves, torn	1 tsp. Himalayan or Celtic sea salt
1 small clove garlic	⅛ tsp. freshly ground black pepper

1. In a high-speed blender, combine almond milk, lemon juice, avocado, kale, garlic, red onion, nutritional yeast flakes, Himalayan sea salt, and black pepper.

2. Blend until completely smooth.

JUICY FACT

Kale has been cultivated for more than 2,000 years. It's widely recognized as one of the most incredibly nutritious vegetables. It's low in fat, has no cholesterol, but is chock full of healthful antioxidant properties.

Spinach Apple Soup

This slightly sweet yet savory soup is a fresh take on the traditional flavors of Indian cuisine. It's reminiscent of garam masala but is also very lively and leaves a clean taste on your palate.

Yield:	Prep time:	Serving size:
about 2½ cups	20 minutes	2½ cups

Each serving has:		
355 calories	42 g carbohydrates	23 g fat
16 g fiber	5 g protein	119% vitamin A
73% vitamin C	10% calcium	26% magnesium
15% iron	37% potassium	

2 cups fresh spinach leaves	¼ small red onion, peeled (¼ cup)
1 small avocado, pitted and peeled	⅛ tsp. ground cinnamon
1 medium-large green apple of choice, peeled and chopped	1 tsp. fresh lemon juice
	Pinch Himalayan or Celtic sea salt
½ cup filtered water	Pinch freshly ground black pepper

1. In a high-speed blender, combine spinach, avocado, green apple, water, red onion, cinnamon, lemon juice, Himalayan sea salt, and black pepper.

2. Blend until completely smooth.

TANTALIZING TIP

For a chilled version of this soup, refrigerate up to 2 hours before serving. This is a nice variation and perfect on a warm summer day. You can also add more water to thin the soup if you like.

Super Mixed Green Salad

Our tangy vinaigrette dressing makes this rainbow salad shine. Tender baby spinach and crunchy lettuce are the perfect bed for crisp cucumber, silky avocado, tart tomato, and sweet bits of carrot.

Yield:	Prep time:	Serving size:
about 4 cups	30 minutes	about 2 cups

Each serving has:		
226 calories	16 g carbohydrates	18 g fat
9 g fiber	4 g protein	304% vitamin A
66% vitamin C	8% calcium	16% magnesium
12% iron	31% potassium	

3 medium romaine lettuce leaves, torn (1 cup)

3 medium red leaf lettuce leaves, torn (1 cup)

1 cup fresh baby spinach

1 small avocado, pitted, peeled, and cubed

⅓ medium cucumber, thinly sliced

¼ large carrot, grated or thinly sliced

½ cup clover sprouts

4 cherry tomatoes, halved

2 TB. dulse flakes

1 TB. apple cider vinegar or balsamic vinegar

½ tsp. Dijon mustard

⅛ tsp. Himalayan or Celtic sea salt

1 TB. cold-pressed extra-virgin olive oil

Pinch freshly ground black pepper

1. In a large salad bowl, combine romaine lettuce, red leaf lettuce, baby spinach, avocado, cucumber, carrot, clover sprouts, cherry tomatoes, and dulse flakes. Set aside.

2. In a high-speed blender or mini food processor, combine apple cider vinegar, Dijon mustard, Himalayan sea salt, and extra-virgin olive oil. Blend until completely smooth.

3. Pour dressing over salad ingredients and toss to coat. Sprinkle with black pepper, and serve immediately.

Avocado Kale Salad

This Asian salad has a tart and mildly cheesy flavor and an amazing mouthfeel that will satisfy any cravings for a heavy meal.

Yield:	Prep time:	Serving size:
about 6 cups	15 minutes	3 cups

Each serving has:		
284 calories	32 g carbohydrates	16 g fat
13 g fiber	12 g protein	528% vitamin A
383% vitamin C	25% calcium	27% magnesium
22% iron	40% potassium	

10 medium-large leaves lacinato kale, finely chopped (5 cups)	½ tsp. Himalayan or Celtic sea salt
1 medium-large avocado, peeled, pitted, and cubed	1 TB. nutritional yeast flakes
Juice of 1 medium lemon	2 medium-large tomatoes, chopped

1. Place chopped lacinato kale in a large salad bowl. Add avocado, and massage avocado into kale, being sure to coat all leaves thoroughly.

2. Sprinkle lemon juice, Himalayan sea salt, and nutritional yeast flakes over salad, and continue massaging until well combined.

3. Gently mix in tomatoes. Serve immediately or allow to marinate at room temperature for about 15 minutes.

JUICY FACT

Avocado kale salads are extremely popular in raw food restaurants all over the world because they're hearty and rich in nutrients. You'll love every bite of this flavorful and satisfying salad.

Raw Waldorf Salad

The Waldorf salad was first created between 1893 and 1896 at the Waldorf Hotel in New York City. This fresh and crunchy raw version will knock your socks off with its complex, sweet, and savory bits.

Yield: 7 cups	Prep time: 20 minutes	Serving size: 2 cups
Each serving has:		
584 calories	95 g carbohydrates	25 g fat
12 g fiber	7 g protein	78% vitamin A
141% vitamin C	11% calcium	23% magnesium
13% iron	49% potassium	

2 medium Fuji apples, diced	¼ cup fresh chives, finely chopped
3 large celery stalks, diced (about 1 cup)	1 medium carrot, grated (¼ cup)
½ cup golden raisins, soaked in 1 cup filtered water for 2 or 3 hours and drained	1 TB. sweet mustard, or 1 tsp. dried mustard seeds
¼ cup dried juice-sweetened cranberries	2 TB. apple cider vinegar
½ large pineapple, peeled, cored, and chopped (2 cups)	2 TB. cold-pressed extra-virgin olive oil
½ cup green grapes, halved	2 medjool dates, pitted
½ cup plus 2 TB. walnuts, crushed	1 tsp. Himalayan or Celtic sea salt
	1 or 2 TB. filtered water

1. In a large salad bowl, combine apples, celery, golden raisins, cranberries, pineapple, green grapes, ½ cup walnuts, chives, and carrot. Set aside.

2. In a high-speed blender or mini food processor, combine remaining 2 tablespoons walnuts, sweet mustard, apple cider vinegar, extra-virgin olive oil, medjool dates, Himalayan sea salt, and water. Blend until completely smooth.

3. Pour dressing over salad, mix until well coated, and serve.

Raw Nori Submarine Sandwich

This raw hero sandwich is bursting with gourmet flavor. You can eat one of these every day and meet most of your nutritional requirements. It's extremely nourishing and absolutely delicious.

Yield:	Prep time:	Serving size:
1 sandwich	20 minutes	1 sandwich

Each serving has:		
479 calories	55 g carbohydrates	31 g fat
21 g fiber	8 g protein	176% vitamin A
318% vitamin C	10% calcium	29% magnesium
17% iron	56% potassium	

1 sheet raw sushi nori

1 large romaine lettuce leaf

1 small tomato, sliced lengthwise

1 small cucumber, sliced into spears

½ small red bell pepper, stem and seeds removed, and sliced into spears

1 medium-small avocado, pitted, peeled, and sliced lengthwise

1 small mango, pitted, peeled, and sliced lengthwise

¼ cup fresh cilantro, chopped fine

⅛ cup mixed greens

⅛ cup sunflower sprouts

Juice of ½ small lemon

Pinch Himalayan or Celtic sea salt

1. Lay nori sheet on a counter. Top with romaine lettuce leaf. Gently arrange tomato slices, cucumber spears, red bell pepper spears, avocado slices, and mango slices on top of romaine lettuce.

2. Add mixed greens and sunflower sprouts, drizzle with lemon juice, and sprinkle with Himalayan sea salt.

3. Dab open end of nori sheet with lemon juice, and gently roll nori into a submarine wrap. Use more lemon juice to help seal nori once rolled together.

4. Cut nori sub in ½, and serve.

Avocado Boats

These avocado boats are terrific as a snack or a meal. They're cheesy, filling, and simple—and highly addictive! Kids love them, too (maybe without the cayenne), so serve up a plate for the whole family.

Yield:	Prep time:	Serving size:
6 avocado boats	15 minutes	1 avocado boat

Each serving has:		
183 calories	11 g carbohydrates	15 g fat
9 g fiber	6 g protein	3% vitamin A
17% vitamin C	1% calcium	10% magnesium
5% iron	14% potassium	

3 medium-large avocados, pitted	2 TB. nutritional yeast flakes
½ tsp. Himalayan or Celtic sea salt	Pinch cayenne
	½ tsp. nama shoyu (optional)

1. Peel avocados, slice in ½, and remove pits.

2. Sprinkle Himalayan sea salt, nutritional yeast flakes, and cayenne into hollow of each ½.

3. Sprinkle nama shoyu (if using) over each avocado boat, and serve.

TANTALIZING TIP

Avocados do not ripen on the tree. They soften after they've been harvested. When choosing an avocado, remember that ripe avocados yield to firm but gentle pressure.

No Bean Raw Hummus

This pungent yet light and zesty hummus spread is complex and delicious. You can use it as a spread in a collard green wrap, add it to a sandwich, or serve it as a dip with some sliced veggies.

Yield:	Prep time:	Serving size:
about 3 cups	15 minutes	½ cup

Each serving has:		
258 calories	12 g carbohydrates	23 g fat
4 g fiber	6 g protein	4% vitamin A
32% vitamin C	14% calcium	11% magnesium
6% iron	11% potassium	

3 medium zucchini, peeled and chopped	2 to 4 small cloves garlic, peeled
¾ cup raw tahini	2½ tsp. Himalayan or Celtic sea salt
¼ cup cold-pressed extra-virgin olive oil	2 tsp. ground cumin
Juice of 1 small lemon	

1. In a high-speed blender, combine zucchini, tahini, extra-virgin olive oil, lemon juice, garlic, Himalayan sea salt, and cumin.

2. Blend until completely smooth.

3. Serve with sliced vegetables such as cucumber, carrots, and zucchini, or roll into a sandwich with 1 collard green. Top with sliced tomato, cucumber, red bell pepper, and/or alfalfa sprouts as desired.

TANTALIZING TIP

When making this recipe, be sure to add the lemon juice and garlic gradually to taste. That way, you can balance the flavors as you like.

Fabulous Fruit Juices

In This Chapter

- Cleansing fruit-juice cocktails
- Fruit-juice recipes to soothe your cravings
- Tropical blends with an exotic flare
- Simple, classic fruit juices

Fruit juices are incredibly cleansing. In general, the sugar content in these juices speed metabolism and tone your tissues, which aids in the release of toxins. They're also an incredible source of healing antioxidants and enzymes. Drink a delicious fruit juice during your prefast days to kick-start your cleansing or anytime you want to give your metabolism a boost and your taste buds a treat.

We highly recommend using organic produce for your juices and leaving on any edible peels. In many fruits, the skin is where the majority of the antioxidant content is stored—hence the red color of apple and grape skins. So leave on those organic skins for some seriously healing phytochemicals.

Pineapple Grape Ginger Juice

You won't believe how delicious this juice tastes! Somehow, it tastes like Lemon Drop candy you might have had as a kid. It's the perfect balance of sweet and tart.

Yield:	Prep time:	Serving size:
about 4 cups	15 minutes	4 cups

Each serving has:		
525 calories	111 g carbohydrates	1 g fat
5 g fiber	5 g protein	11% vitamin A
559% vitamin C	11% calcium	24% magnesium
16% iron	35% potassium	

3 cups red grapes	1 (½-in.) piece peeled fresh ginger
1 medium pineapple, peeled, cored, and sliced	

1. In a low-rpm juicer, alternate pressing red grapes, pineapple slices, and ginger.

2. Stir and serve immediately.

PULPY PITFALL

This delicious juice is a vitamin C powerhouse that improves digestion and kidney function, helps regulate blood sugar, and gives you an overall immune system boost. But please note that this juice uses a lot of pineapple, which is brimming with healing compounds but can be irritating if taken too often. We recommend drinking this juice no more than three times a week during your cleanse.

Red Grape Strawberry Juice

This mildly sweet and fruity juice is reminiscent of a strawberry icicle pop. The taste is smooth, and you'll be tempted to drink it quickly. But restrain yourself, and savor each drop.

Yield:	Prep time:	Serving size:
about 4 cups	15 minutes	4 cups

Each serving has:		
596 calories	147 g carbohydrates	1 g fat
8 g fiber	6 g protein	11% vitamin A
401% vitamin C	12% calcium	22% magnesium
21% iron	53% potassium	

2 medium-large bunches red grapes (about 5 cups)	15 medium-large strawberries, green leaves intact

1. In a low-rpm juicer, alternate pressing red grapes and strawberries.

2. Stir and serve immediately.

JUICY FACT

Grapes and strawberries are incredibly healthful. Grapes offer protection from heart disease and incredible anticancer properties, and both grapes and strawberries give you a surge of powerful antioxidants.

Apple Pear Lemon Juice

A wonderful combination of sweet, sour, and tangy, this juice is very refreshing and has an almost sparkling sensation as you drink it.

Yield:	Prep time:	Serving size:
about 4 cups	15 minutes	4 cups

Each serving has:		
589 calories	122 g carbohydrates	2 g fat
6 g fiber	3 g protein	9% vitamin A
131% vitamin C	10% calcium	19% magnesium
11% iron	38% potassium	

3 medium red apples, cored and sliced	1 small lemon, outer rind removed, white pith intact
3 medium pears, cored and sliced	1 (2-in.) piece peeled fresh ginger

1. In a low-rpm juicer, alternate pressing red apple slices, pear slices, lemon, and ginger.

2. Stir and serve immediately.

JUICY FACT

This is a perfect juice to drink during the winter when other produce is scarce. It's also great for preventing high blood pressure, lowering cholesterol, regulating bowel movements, providing increased energy, and preventing osteoporosis.

Cantaloupe Juice

This incredibly filling juice has a unique, fruity, sweet flavor with a surprisingly creamy texture. A real taste-bud sensation, this juice will fulfill your cravings for sweets during your cleanse.

Yield:	Prep time:	Serving size:
about 4 cups	15 minutes	4 cups

Each serving has:		
365 calories	87 g carbohydrates	2 g fat
5 g fiber	7 g protein	747% vitamin A
675% vitamin C	10% calcium	33% magnesium
13% iron	84% potassium	

> 2 medium cantaloupes, coarse outer rind removed, inner green rind intact, seeded, and sliced

1. In a low-rpm juicer, press cantaloupe slices.

2. Stir and serve immediately.

JUICY FACT

Cantaloupes are the most nutritious fruit on the planet. They offer protection for your immune system as well as ample anticancer properties. They also help improve your eyesight, prevent hardening of the arteries, and decrease anxiety and insomnia by toning the nervous system.

Orange Grapefruit Strawberry Juice

This delicious and energizing juice has a classic tart citrus twist that pairs with just the right balance of sweetness and berry flavor. Its amazing zing will keep you coming back for more.

Yield:	Prep time:	Serving size:
about 4 cups	15 minutes	4 cups

Each serving has:		
370 calories	66 g carbohydrates	1 g fat
4 g fiber	8 g protein	112% vitamin A
693% vitamin C	22% calcium	23% magnesium
7% iron	44% potassium	

2 medium grapefruits, outer rind peeled, white pith intact, and sectioned

2 medium navel oranges, outer rind peeled, white pith intact, and sectioned

5 or 6 large fresh strawberries, green leaves intact

1. In a low-rpm juicer, alternate pressing grapefruit sections, orange sections, and strawberries.

2. Stir and serve immediately.

TANTALIZING TIP

When choosing your grapefruit, heavier is better and means there's lots of juice inside. Drink grapefruit juice often for the protection it offers from colon and lung cancer, and for its ample supply of antioxidants.

Lemon Apple Juice

Soothing and refreshing, this juice tastes like a sweet, mild lemonade.

Yield:	Prep time:	Serving size:
about 4 cups	15 minutes	4 cups

Each serving has:		
563 calories	120 g carbohydrates	2 g fat
7 g fiber	3 g protein	12% vitamin A
158% vitamin C	9% calcium	15% magnesium
10% iron	37% potassium	

6 medium Fuji apples, cored and sliced	1 large lemon, outer rind peeled, white pith intact, and sectioned

1. In a low-rpm juicer, alternate pressing Fuji apple slices with lemon sections.

2. Stir and serve immediately.

JUICY FACT

Apple juices are wonderful because they contain soluble fiber, which isn't removed during the juicing process. Drink this juice, and others containing apple, often during your juice fast to help cleanse your digestive system.

Honeydew Lime Juice

Tantalizingly sweet with a bright and zingy finish, this creamy juice tastes like a mild tropical hard candy.

Yield:	Prep time:	Serving size:
about 4 cups	15 minutes	4 cups

Each serving has:		
352 calories	80 g carbohydrates	1 g fat
3 g fiber	5 g protein	11% vitamin A
333% vitamin C	8% calcium	26% magnesium
12% iron	67% potassium	

2 medium-small honeydew melons outer rind peeled, inner rind intact, seeded, and sliced	1 small lime, outer rind peeled, white pith intact

1. In a low-rpm juicer, alternate pressing honeydew melon slices and lime.

2. Stir and serve immediately.

TANTALIZING TIP

When choosing your honeydew, look for melons that are slightly soft and have a creamy yellow navel. Harder melons won't be sweet and do not ripen off the vine. Also smell the melon before buying. Ripe melons are very aromatic.

Pineapple Strawberry Juice

This juice has a stimulating tropical taste. Pineapple and strawberry create a synergistic flavor combination that's both mildly tart and syrupy sweet.

Yield:	Prep time:	Serving size:
about 4 cups	15 minutes	4 cups

Each serving has:		
487 calories	112 g carbohydrates	2 g fat
7 g fiber	6 g protein	11% vitamin A
897% vitamin C	15% calcium	33% magnesium
19% iron	36% potassium	

1 large pineapple, peeled, cored, and sliced	8 to 10 medium-large strawberries, green leaves intact

1. In a low-rpm juicer, alternate pressing pineapple slices and strawberries.

2. Stir and serve immediately.

JUICY FACT

This powerful and healthy juice will flush any excess mucus out of your body. Its anti-inflammatory properties heal digestive disorders and improve cold and detox symptoms.

Pear Apple Ginger Juice

This delicious juice combination is sweet with just enough of a spicy bite to excite your taste buds. It'll put a zip in your step to keep you going on your juice fast.

Yield:	Prep time:	Serving size:
about 4 cups	15 minutes	4 cups

Each serving has:		
583 calories	130 g carbohydrates	1 g fat
10 g fiber	4 g protein	7% vitamin A
78% vitamin C	9% calcium	18% magnesium
9% iron	36% potassium	

4 medium pears, cored and sliced	1 (1-in.) piece peeled fresh ginger
2 medium Granny Smith apples, cored and sliced	

1. In a low-rpm juicer, alternate pressing pear slices, Granny Smith apple slices, and ginger.

2. Stir and serve immediately.

JUICY FACT

This juice protects against brain aging, reduces the risk of cancer, relieves constipation, lowers cholesterol levels, and is an amazing colon cleanser. It'll really clean out your entire system.

Lime Orange Juice

This sweet and tangy juice gives your taste buds an amazing fruity citrus punch.

Yield:	Prep time:	Serving size:
about 4 cups	15 minutes	4 cups

Each serving has:		
476 calories	98 g carbohydrates	3 g fat
5 g fiber	10 g protein	45% vitamin A
815% vitamin C	41% calcium	25% magnesium
7% iron	51% potassium	

5 medium navel oranges, outer rind peeled, white pith intact, and sectioned	1 small lime, outer rind peeled, white pith intact

1. In a low-rpm juicer, alternate pressing orange sections and lime.

2. Stir and serve immediately.

TANTALIZING TIP

When choosing limes, pick fruits that are dark green and heavy. Dark-colored limes have the most distinctive lime flavor. Avoid limes with purple or brown spots.

Cranberry Pear Juice

This sweet and super-tart juice will knock your socks off! It's a perfect cleansing cocktail with a beautiful glowing red hue.

Yield:	Prep time:	Serving size:
about 4 cups	15 minutes	4 cups

Each serving has:		
685 calories	140 g carbohydrates	2 g fat
11 g fiber	5 g protein	7% vitamin A
119% vitamin C	11% calcium	22% magnesium
13% iron	41% potassium	

6 medium-large pears, cored and sliced	2 cups fresh cranberries

1. In a low-rpm juicer, alternate pressing pear slices and cranberries.

2. Stir and serve immediately.

JUICY FACT

Cranberries are amazing for toning the kidneys and clearing up a troubled complexion. Combined with fresh apple juice, cranberries become a cleansing powerhouse for balancing blood sugar and opening your detoxification channels.

Orange Juice

This juice will blow your mind. Compared to this drink, your typical fresh-squeezed orange juice tastes like sugar water. This juice recalls a creamsicle ice-pop you may remember from childhood.

Yield:	Prep time:	Serving size:
about 4 cups	15 minutes	4 cups

Each serving has:		
452 calories	99 g carbohydrates	1 g fat
4 g fiber	7 g protein	48% vitamin A
965% vitamin C	42% calcium	27% magnesium
7% iron	46% potassium	

8 medium-large navel oranges, outer rind peeled, white pith intact, and sectioned

1. In a low-rpm juicer, press orange sections.

2. Stir and serve immediately.

TANTALIZING TIP

When you prepare any citrus fruits for juicing, do your best to leave as much of the white pith on as possible. The pith is packed with phytonutrients like bioflavonoids. This juicy taste sensation boosts your immune system, increases iron absorption, prevents skin cancer (melanoma), and reduces low-density lipoprotein (bad cholesterol).

Apple Orange Juice

This wonderful juice combination gives you a burst of mouthwatering flavor. The sweet apple balances the slight tartness of the orange perfectly.

Yield:	Prep time:	Serving size:
about 4 cups	15 minutes	4 cups

Each serving has:		
574 calories	124 g carbohydrates	3 g fat
9 g fiber	6 g protein	30% vitamin A
447% vitamin C	24% calcium	21% magnesium
7% iron	47% potassium	

4 medium red apples, cored and sliced	4 medium Valencia oranges, outer rind peeled, white pith intact, and sectioned

1. In a low-rpm juicer, alternate pressing red apple slices and orange sections.

2. Stir and serve immediately.

JUICY FACT

This juice provides an incredible amount of disease-fighting antioxidants and is loaded with vitamin C. It also lowers hypertension and reduces inflammation.

Watermelon Juice

This juice tastes like a mild version of a classic watermelon candy you may have enjoyed as a child. The slightly sweet taste and subtly creamy texture are so delicious.

Yield:	Prep time:	Serving size:
about 4 cups	15 minutes	4 cups

Each serving has:		
316 calories	80 g carbohydrates	2 g fat
1 g fiber	6 g protein	129% vitamin A
152% vitamin C	8% calcium	28% magnesium
15% iron	36% potassium	

1 medium-large seeded watermelon, outer skin peeled, inner rind intact, and sliced

1. In a low-rpm juicer, press watermelon slices.

2. Stir and serve immediately.

JUICY FACT

In addition to tasting great, this juice provides incredible anti-aging benefits. It's loaded with antioxidants and other phytonutrients that protect against stomach, lung, and prostate cancer. This tasty drink is also a powerful diuretic that flushes your system very efficiently.

Apple Ginger Juice

This incredible juice is super sweet with a slightly spicy zip that will jump-start your day.

Yield:	Prep time:	Serving size:
about 4 cups	15 minutes	4 cups

Each serving has:		
1,124 calories	132 g carbohydrates	2 g fat
9 g fiber	4 g protein	14% vitamin A
99% vitamin C	8% calcium	17% magnesium
9% iron	40% potassium	

7 medium Fuji or green apples, cored and sliced	1 (2-in.) piece peeled fresh ginger

1. In a low-rpm juicer, alternate pressing Fuji apple slices and ginger.

2. Stir and serve immediately.

TANTALIZING TIP

This juice is an excellent tonic for cold and flu prevention. It provides migraine relief and general pain alleviation, thanks to its anti-inflammatory effect. It's also known as a colon cancer preventative.

Pomegranate Apple Grape Juice

In this velvety sweet juice, pomegranate and lime spring through the sweet flavor of red grapes with a sharp tartness sure to please any palate.

Yield:	Prep time:	Serving size:
about 4 cups	15 minutes	4 cups

Each serving has:		
686 calories	161 g carbohydrates	4 g fat
8 g fiber	9 g protein	11% vitamin A
177% vitamin C	11% calcium	22% magnesium
17% iron	54% potassium	

1 medium pomegranate	3 cups red grapes
3 medium Fuji apples, cored and sliced	½ medium lime, outer rind peeled, white pith intact, and sectioned

1. Cut pomegranate in half, and scoop out seeds. Using a food mill, grind fresh juice from seeds, leaving seeds trapped in the mill. Alternatively, you can hand press the seeds in a muslin cloth, retaining juice in a bowl.

2. In a low-rpm juicer, alternate pressing Fuji apple slices, red grapes, and lime sections.

3. Gently stir in pomegranate juice.

4. Serve immediately.

PULPY PITFALL

Pomegranates are loaded with healthful antioxidants, but never press your pomegranate seeds through your juicer or you'll end up with an unpleasant-tasting, bitter, astringent juice.

Pineapple Grapefruit Juice

This bittersweet juice has an invigorating tropical taste that gives you the feeling of watching the waves crash on a secluded beach.

Yield:	Prep time:	Serving size:
about 4 cups	15 minutes	4 cups

Each serving has:		
423 calories	102 g carbohydrates	1 g fat
3 g fiber	5 g protein	21% vitamin A
729% vitamin C	13% calcium	27% magnesium
13% iron	31% potassium	

1 medium pineapple, peeled, cored, and sliced	1 medium grapefruit, outer rind peeled, white pith intact, and sectioned

1. In a low-rpm juicer, alternate pressing pineapple slices and grapefruit sections.

2. Stir and serve immediately.

JUICY FACT

This cleansing juice kick-starts your metabolism. It offers amazing protection against cancers of all types and reduces the negative effects of exposure to cigarette smoke.

Tangerine Pineapple Juice

This juice is the epitome of the word *zesty* with its sparks of tangy citrus and sweet pineapple that will wake up your taste buds.

Yield:	Prep time:	Serving size:
about 4 cups	15 minutes	4 cups

Each serving has:		
713 calories	169 g carbohydrates	3 g fat
4 g fiber	10 g protein	104% vitamin A
890% vitamin C	35% calcium	43% magnesium
18% iron	56% potassium	

1 medium pineapple, peeled, cored, and sliced	8 medium tangerines, outer rind peeled, white pith intact, and sectioned

1. In a low-rpm juicer, alternate pressing pineapple slices and tangerine sections.

2. Stir and serve immediately.

TANTALIZING TIP

This scrumptious juice is a fantastic immunity booster, so make it a regular during cold and flu season. This juice can help improve eyesight, thin your blood, relieve arthritis symptoms, and protect you from breast cancer.

Apple Pink Grapefruit Juice

With its delightfully sweet and citrusy sensation, this juice is perfect for both fans and skeptics of grapefruit.

Yield:	Prep time:	Serving size:
about 4 cups	15 minutes	4 cups

Each serving has:		
437 calories	93 g carbohydrates	1 g fat
5 g fiber	3 g protein	21% vitamin A
208% vitamin C	8% calcium	14% magnesium
6% iron	31% potassium	

4 medium Fuji or honeycrisp apples, cored and sliced	1 medium pink grapefruit, outer rind peeled, white pith intact, and sectioned

1. In a low-rpm juicer, alternate pressing Fuji apple slices and pink grapefruit sections.

2. Stir and serve immediately.

TANTALIZING TIP

Drink this juice when you want to feel full. It takes care of any nagging cravings you'll experience during your fast while boosting your metabolism and soothing your entire digestive system.

Kiwi Apple Juice

This super-sweet tropical juice will satisfy your cravings and fulfill any desires you might have for a seriously indulgent dessert.

Yield:	Prep time:	Serving size:
about 4 cups	15 minutes	4 cups

Each serving has:		
677 calories	150 g carbohydrates	3 g fat
4 g fiber	4 g protein	16% vitamin A
436% vitamin C	14% calcium	23% magnesium
11% iron	54% potassium	

6 medium Fuji apples, cored and sliced	4 small kiwis, peeled

1. In a low-rpm juicer, alternate pressing Fuji apple slices and kiwis.

2. Stir and serve immediately.

PULPY PITFALL

This juice contains serious protective elements that promote tissue regeneration and longevity. Kiwis, much like pineapples, are loaded with healing compounds, but can be irritating to your system if taken in large amounts. Moderation is key.

Vivacious Vegetable Juices

In This Chapter

- Tantalizing veggie juices
- Fresh vegetable-and-fruit juices
- Nutritionally powerful vegetable juices

Fresh, raw, organic vegetable juices are an exciting and delicious way to feed your body with essential nutrients only found in the plant kingdom. A necessary component of a successful juice fast, vegetable juices are also an integral part of your overall health regimen. The tasty blends in this chapter are filled with an abundance of leafy greens and vibrant vegetables, all of which are packed with the phytochemicals, antioxidants, vitamins, and minerals that keep your electrolytes balanced and bathe your cells in healing nutrition.

While juice fasting, you may at times experience mild detox symptoms like headaches or flulike feelings. The following nutrient-dense vegetable juices are the perfect way to ease any discomfort while still supporting your cleansing program. They help moderate the detox process and make your cleanse much more pleasant.

For any juice fast lasting longer than 1 day, use these vegetable juices as your mainstay. You may also drink pure fruit juices intermittently throughout the day, but the recipes in this chapter are specifically formulated to provide your body with concentrated nutrition and lasting energy.

Carrot Apple Lemon Juice

Sweet carrots and apples are perfectly balanced with the tang of tart lemon, savory celery, and robust bell pepper.

Yield:	Prep time:	Serving size:
about 4 cups	15 minutes	2 cups
Each serving has:		
248 calories	61 g carbohydrates	1 g fat
4 g fiber	5 g protein	844% vitamin A
209% vitamin C	15% calcium	16% magnesium
10% iron	43% potassium	

6 medium-large carrots

3 medium Fuji apples, cored and sliced

3 large celery stalks

1 medium red bell pepper, stem and seeds removed, and sliced

3 large Romaine lettuce leaves

Juice of 1 medium lemon

1. In a low-rpm juicer, alternate pressing carrots, Fuji apple slices, celery, red bell pepper slices, and Romaine lettuce leaves.

2. Stir in hand-squeezed lemon juice.

3. Serve immediately.

JUICY FACT

This juice detoxifies the liver. Aside from this major benefit, the ingredients in this juice are known for their ability to lower cholesterol, soothe the nervous system, and prevent kidney stones. It's also a strong blood alkalizer that can improve eyesight.

Celery Swiss Chard Kale Juice

This earthy, filling juice is a perfect blend of sweet and savory flavors. It leaves you feeling quite satisfied.

Yield:	Prep time:	Serving size:
about 4 cups	15 minutes	2 cups

Each serving has:		
292 calories	54 g carbohydrates	2 g fat
4 g fiber	12 g protein	1,390% vitamin A
501% vitamin C	46% calcium	53% magnesium
37% iron	70% potassium	

6 medium carrots	2 medium green apples, cored and sliced
4 large celery stalks	6 small Swiss chard leaves
4 medium kale leaves	

1. In a low-rpm juicer, alternate pressing carrots, celery, kale leaves, green apple slices, and Swiss chard leaves.

2. Stir and serve immediately.

JUICY FACT

This detoxifying juice blend reduces the risk of cancer, maintains strong bone density, can reduce the risk of stroke, and ensures proper kidney function.

Cucumber Apple Celery Cilantro Juice

This sweet and slightly spicy juice is tinged with warming ginger and has an aromatic citrus flavor imparted by cilantro, nature's natural *chelator*. It's a real kick for your taste buds.

Yield:	Prep time:	Serving size:
about 4 cups	15 minutes	2 cups

Each serving has:		
161 calories	38 g carbohydrates	1 g fat
3 g fiber	2 g protein	22% vitamin A
34% vitamin C	8% calcium	10% magnesium
5% iron	21% potassium	

1 medium cucumber	3 large celery stalks
3 medium Fuji apples, cored and sliced	5 large sprigs cilantro

1. In a low-rpm juicer, alternate pressing cucumber, Fuji apple slices, celery, and cilantro.

2. Stir and serve immediately.

DEFINITION

A **chelator** is a substance that draws heavy metals, toxic chemicals, and other impurities from your blood and other tissues in your body. After these substances are chelated, they can be removed from your body by its normal cleansing processes.

Carrot Parsley Cabbage Juice

Aromatic parsley makes this sweet and slightly pungent juice tingle on your tongue.

Yield:	Prep time:	Serving size:
about 4 cups	15 minutes	2 cups

Each serving has:		
135 calories	20 g carbohydrates	1 g fat
2 g fiber	5 g protein	849% vitamin A
99% vitamin C	22% calcium	23% magnesium
18% iron	45% potassium	

6 large carrots	3 cups fresh spinach, packed
6 large celery stalks	
¼ medium bunch curly parsley	½ cup chopped green cabbage

1. In a low-rpm juicer, alternate pressing carrots, celery, curly parsley, spinach, and green cabbage.

2. Stir and serve immediately.

JUICY FACT

This powerhouse detox juice is perfect for cleansing, reconstruction, and regeneration of the intestinal tract. It also helps maintain proper adrenal and thyroid gland function.

Apple Dandelion Cilantro Juice

Pungent dandelion greens mix wonderfully into the sweet flavor of apple and the slight citrus undertones of lively cilantro.

Yield:	Prep time:	Serving size:
about 4 cups	15 minutes	2 cups

Each serving has:		
246 calories	55 g carbohydrates	1 g fat
5 g fiber	3 g protein	89% vitamin A
64% vitamin C	15% calcium	13% magnesium
11% iron	30% potassium	

5 medium Fuji apples, cored and sliced	5 large celery stalks
6 large dandelion greens	½ cup fresh cilantro, chopped

1. In a low-rpm juicer, alternate pressing Fuji apple slices, dandelion greens, celery, and cilantro.

2. Stir and serve immediately.

JUICY FACT

This juice is a great source of organic magnesium, one of the most potent healing juices on the planet. It gives your teeth and gums strength and density, and your body uses it to manufacture calcium. It also relaxes tense or strained muscles.

Cucumber Beet Carrot Juice

Mildly sweet and incredibly thirst quenching, this juice has a full and rich, savory flavor.

Yield:	Prep time:	Serving size:
about 4 cups	15 minutes	2 cups

Each serving has:		
179 calories	39 g carbohydrates	1 g fat
3 g fiber	7 g protein	1,287% vitamin A
73% vitamin C	21% calcium	28% magnesium
18% iron	57% potassium	

12 medium carrots	1 large red beet
1 medium-large cucumber	3 medium beet greens

1. In a low-rpm juicer, alternate pressing carrots, cucumber, red beet, and beet greens.

2. Stir and serve immediately.

TANTALIZING TIP

This is one of the most detoxifying juices you can drink. It also tastes great, so you might find yourself craving it when your body needs a quick detox. This is a perfect juice to drink regularly throughout your juice fast or as a part of your daily health program.

Lettuce Apple Celery Carrot Juice

This mild-flavored juice is a cleansing powerhouse! Sweet and delicious, it's also very healing and purifying.

Yield:	Prep time:	Serving size:
about 4 cups	15 minutes	2 cups

Each serving has:		
230 calories	50 g carbohydrates	1 g fat
5 g fiber	4 g protein	808% vitamin A
88% vitamin C	15% calcium	15% magnesium
12% iron	40% potassium	

5 large carrots	4 large romaine lettuce leaves
3 medium Fuji apples, cored and sliced	4 large red leaf lettuce leaves
3 large celery stalks	

1. In a low-rpm juicer, alternate pressing carrots, Fuji apple slices, celery, romaine lettuce leaves, and red leaf lettuce leaves.

2. Stir and serve immediately.

JUICY FACT

This cleansing juice has exceptional vitalizing powers, particularly in the muscular tissues, brain, and nervous system. This juice combination is a perfect tonic to encourage the growth of hair and restore graying hair to its natural color.

Cucumber Beet Coconut Juice

With a slightly tropical twist, this sweet juice has a deeply satisfying mild and clean taste.

Yield:	Prep time:	Serving size:
about 4 cups	15 minutes	2 cups

Each serving has:		
98 calories	16 g carbohydrates	1 g fat
1 g fiber	5 g protein	67% vitamin A
50% vitamin C	17% calcium	35% magnesium
17% iron	43% potassium	

2 medium-large cucumbers	3 medium beet greens
½ large red beet, chopped	Water from 1 large young coconut (2 cups)

1. In a low-rpm juicer, alternate pressing cucumbers, red beet, and beet greens.

2. Stir in young coconut water.

3. Serve immediately.

JUICY FACT

This juice is not only cleansing, it's an incredible body builder. It has potent kidney- and gall bladder–cleansing properties and also gives you extra energy during your cleansing program.

Carrot Parsley Beet Juice

This sweet and earthy juice is the perfect carrier for aromatic and herbal parsley.

Yield:	Prep time:	Serving size:
about 4 cups	15 minutes	2 cups
Each serving has:		
209 calories	35 g carbohydrates	1 g fat
2 g fiber	7 g protein	1,598% vitamin A
86% vitamin C	22% calcium	27% magnesium
19% iron	59% potassium	

15 medium carrots	3 medium beet greens
1 large red beet, chopped	6 large sprigs curly parsley

1. In a low-rpm juicer, alternate pressing carrots, red beet, beet greens, and curly parsley.

2. Stir and serve immediately.

PULPY PITFALL

This juice is extremely beneficial to the liver and gall bladder. It's well known for building up the red corpuscles and stimulating activity of the lymphatic system throughout the entire body. But be aware that beet greens and beets contain oxalic acid, which can exacerbate arthritis and some other inflammatory diseases.

Apple Ginger Parsley Carrot Juice

Sweet with a warm, gingery kick and the zest of fresh herbal parsley, this juice is the definition of *vital!*

Yield:	Prep time:	Serving size:
about 4 cups	15 minutes	2 cups
Each serving has:		
250 calories	55 g carbohydrates	1 g fat
3 g fiber	4 g protein	974% vitamin A
61% vitamin C	12% calcium	23% magnesium
8% iron	36% potassium	

8 large carrots

3 medium Fuji apples, cored and sliced

1 (½-in.) piece peeled fresh ginger

5 large sprigs curly parsley

1. In a low-rpm juicer, alternate pressing carrots, Fuji apple slices, ginger, and curly parsley.

2. Stir and serve immediately.

JUICY FACT

This detoxifying juice lowers cholesterol and is incredible for improving your immune system function while you're fighting off a cold.

Gorgeous Green Juices

In This Chapter

- Great-tasting green juice blends
- Electrolyte-balancing juices
- Juices packed with the healing properties of leafy greens

Green juices are an essential component of a successful juice fast. Chlorophyll-rich dark-green leaves alkalize the blood and neutralize free radicals in your body. The structure of chlorophyll is almost identical to the hemoglobin in human blood, which is responsible for carrying oxygen to your cells.

Juicing greens is a great way to work more of them into your diet and in a very enjoyable way. In this chapter, you'll find green juices that appeal to anyone's taste buds. Some are sweet, some are sour, and others are mild and earthy. The juice combinations are well varied and will make converts out of anyone who claims they "don't like greens."

Make green juices a part of your daily juice-fasting regimen to ensure you're getting the best nutrition possible along with superior cleansing power.

Celery Cucumber Kale Chard Parsley Juice

This juice is wonderfully grounding. It has a mild herbal flavor that complements its smooth sweetness. This juice makes a perfect mid-day snack during your juice fast.

Yield:	Prep time:	Serving size:
about 4 cups	15 minutes	4 cups

Each serving has:		
483 calories	86 g carbohydrates	4 g fat
7 g fiber	14 g protein	1,029% vitamin A
680% vitamin C	54% calcium	69% magnesium
50% iron	82% potassium	

1 large celery stalk	4 medium kale leaves
1 medium-large cucumber, sliced	3 medium chard leaves
3 medium Granny Smith apples, cored and sliced	5 large sprigs parsley

1. In a low-rpm juicer, alternate pressing celery, cucumber, green apple slices, kale leaves, chard leaves, and parsley.

2. Stir and serve immediately.

JUICY FACT

This juice is a nutrition powerhouse. Some of its health benefits include protection from coronary artery disease, reduced risk of cancer and stroke, and improved eyesight.

Celery Green Apple Spinach Juice

This is a simple and refreshing juice. Its sweet, earthy flavor is the epitome of a fresh and mild juice anyone can enjoy.

Yield:	Prep time:	Serving size:
about 4 cups	15 minutes	4 cups

Each serving has:		
532 calories	123 g carbohydrates	3 g fat
10 g fiber	10 g protein	468% vitamin A
188% vitamin C	34% calcium	62% magnesium
43% iron	75% potassium	

2 large celery stalks	1 medium bunch spinach
5 medium Granny Smith apples, cored and sliced	

1. In a low-rpm juicer, alternate pressing celery, green apple slices, and spinach.

2. Stir and serve immediately.

TANTALIZING TIP

This is a delicious postworkout juice that provides incredible electrolyte replenishment. The sodium-potassium balance is perfect to drink after a morning exercise routine to stave off sore muscles or cramps and fatigue. Its mineral density can also help relieve migraine headaches and support a healthy cardiovascular system.

Apple Collard Kale Cilantro Juice

This robust juice is sweet, savory, and fresh with a slight citrus/basil flavor thanks to fresh cilantro.

Yield:	Prep time:	Serving size:
about 4 cups	15 minutes	4 cups

Each serving has:		
568 calories	113 g carbohydrates	3 g fat
9 g fiber	10 g protein	593% vitamin A
410% vitamin C	41% calcium	26% magnesium
22% iron	53% potassium	

5 medium Fuji apples, cored and sliced

3 medium collard green leaves

3 medium kale leaves

6 to 8 large sprigs cilantro

1. In a low-rpm juicer, alternate pressing Fuji apple slices, collard greens, kale leaves, and cilantro.

2. Stir and serve immediately.

JUICY FACT

This juice is revered for its nutritional and medicinal qualities. It boasts many healing benefits, builds bone density, and strengthens the kidneys. It also offers valued protection from colon cancer and cataracts.

Celery Cucumber Lemon Apple Kale Ginger Juice

This zesty, sweet, and sour juice is full-flavored with just the right blend of bright, light flavors and a mild spicy kick. The ginger and lemon are delightful.

Yield:	Prep time:	Serving size:
about 4 cups	15 minutes	4 cups

Each serving has:		
401 calories	87 g carbohydrates	2 g fat
6 g fiber	8 g protein	430% vitamin A
377% vitamin C	30% calcium	30% magnesium
23% iron	53% potassium	

2 medium celery stalks

1 medium cucumber, sliced

1 medium lemon, outer rind removed, white pith intact, and sectioned

3 medium Granny Smith apples, cored and chopped

3 large kale leaves

1 (1-in.) piece peeled fresh ginger

1. In a low-rpm juicer, alternate pressing celery, cucumber, lemon sections, Granny Smith apple slices, kale leaves, and ginger.

2. Stir and serve immediately.

TANTALIZING TIP

This juice is extremely detoxifying and will really amp up your cleanse. Drink this anytime you need to dissolve mucous from a cold. It will totally scour toxins from your cellular tissue while opening elimination channels.

Spinach Celery Apple Cucumber Collard Juice

This flavorful juice has a well balanced taste with slightly sweet, mellow, and earthy flavors. You'll feel refreshed and nourished after just one glass.

Yield:	Prep time:	Serving size:
about 4 cups	15 minutes	4 cups

Each serving has:		
427 calories	83 g carbohydrates	3 g fat
8 g fiber	13 g protein	640% vitamin A
254% vitamin C	43% calcium	99% magnesium
60% iron	92% potassium	

3 medium celery stalks	2 medium cucumbers, sliced
3 medium Fuji apples, cored and sliced	4 medium chard leaves
1 medium bunch spinach	1 (1-in.) piece peeled fresh ginger

1. In a low-rpm juicer, alternate pressing celery, Fuji apple slices, spinach, cucumbers, chard leaves, and ginger.

2. Stir and serve immediately.

TANTALIZING TIP

This juice enhances the suppleness of your skin and will make your hair and nails shine, so drink it anytime to help clear up your complexion. It's an incredible anti-aging drink that derives its power from its diuretic action as it flushes waste from your system and allows your skin to heal.

Romaine Celery Kale Pear Lemon Juice

This flavorful juice has a mellow taste that's savory, delicately sweet, and just a bit zingy.

Yield:	Prep time:	Serving size:
about 4 cups	15 minutes	4 cups

Each serving has:		
563 calories	119 g carbohydrates	4 g fat
11 g fiber	16 g protein	1,543% vitamin A
989% vitamin C	72% calcium	55% magnesium
56% iron	94% potassium	

3 medium pears, cored
  and sliced

2 large celery stalks

6 medium kale leaves

1 medium lemon, outer
  rind removed, white
  pith intact, and
  sectioned

6 medium romaine
  lettuce leaves

1. In a low-rpm juicer, alternate pressing pear slices, celery, kale leaves, lemon sections, and romaine lettuce leaves.

2. Stir and serve immediately.

JUICY FACT

This juice is extremely cleansing and will help clean out your digestive system. It's a natural body deodorizer and supports the production of hemoglobin. Drink this juice often for the protection it offers against brain aging, cancer, and high cholesterol.

Cucumber Lemon Kale Juice

This subtle juice has a neutral flavor with a tart and tangy twist that makes it lively and fresh tasting.

Yield:	Prep time:	Serving size:
about 4 cups	15 minutes	4 cups

Each serving has:		
276 calories	46 g carbohydrates	3 g fat
5 g fiber	13 g protein	1,045% vitamin A
776% vitamin C	58% calcium	53% magnesium
45% iron	75% potassium	

3 medium-large cucumbers, sliced	1 medium lemon, outer rind removed, white pith intact, and sectioned
5 medium kale leaves	

1. In a low-rpm juicer, alternate pressing cucumbers, kale leaves, and lemon sections.

2. Stir and serve immediately.

JUICY FACT

This juice helps protect against coronary artery disease and lowers the risk of stroke and kidney problems. It also improves your eyesight and helps clear up skin blemishes.

Cabbage Cucumber Spinach Kale Juice

This juice tastes fresh, flavorful, and mild. Cabbage adds a slightly sweet and zesty taste that blends nicely with the other ingredients for an earthy and smooth finish.

Yield:	Prep time:	Serving size:
about 4 cups	15 minutes	4 cups

Each serving has:		
359 calories	73 g carbohydrates	3 g fat
7 g fiber	13 g protein	686% vitamin A
520% vitamin C	43% calcium	45% magnesium
35% iron	66% potassium	

2 medium-large cucumbers, sliced	Large handful fresh spinach leaves
3 large kale leaves	½ very small head cabbage, chopped (about 1 cup)
2 medium Fuji apples, cored and sliced	

1. In a low-rpm juicer, alternate pressing cucumbers, kale leaves, Fuji apple slices, spinach leaves, and cabbage.

2. Stir and serve immediately.

JUICY FACT

This juice has an amazing ability to heal digestive disorders. It's also chock full of phytonutrients that protect against lung, breast, prostate, and colon cancers.

Kale Mustard Red Grape Lemon Juice

This juice is a zinger, with its potent sweet taste and stimulating, spicy and zesty taste sensation.

Yield:	Prep time:	Serving size:
about 4 cups	15 minutes	4 cups

Each serving has:		
547 calories	126 g carbohydrates	3 g fat
3 g fiber	13 g protein	850% vitamin A
729% vitamin C	45% calcium	36% magnesium
41% iron	71% potassium	

2 medium-large bunches red grapes (4 cups)	1 medium lemon, outer rind removed, white pith intact, and sectioned
4 medium kale leaves	1 small mustard green leaf

1. In a low-rpm juicer, alternate pressing red grapes, kale leaves, lemon sections, and mustard green leaf.

2. Stir and serve immediately.

PULPY PITFALL

Mustard greens contain volatile oils that give them their characteristic spiciness. Raw mustard greens add a flavor somewhat similar to wasabi, although far milder. Just be careful not to overdo it on these potent healing greens; a little goes a long way!

Celery Wheatgrass Juice

This juice has an earthy yet supremely sweet taste that works perfectly with zingy lemon. The combination creates a delicious and palatable drink that even makes wheatgrass juice enjoyable.

Yield:	Prep time:	Serving size:
about 4 cups	15 minutes	4 cups

Each serving has:		
431 calories	97 g carbohydrates	2 g fat
9 g fiber	5 g protein	31% vitamin A
135% vitamin C	16% calcium	17% magnesium
30% iron	44% potassium	

3 bunches wheatgrass (2 oz.)	1 medium lemon, outer rind removed, white pith intact, and sectioned
4 large celery stalks	4 medium Fuji apples, cored and sliced

1. In a low-rpm juicer, alternate pressing wheatgrass, celery, lemon sections, and Fuji apple slices.

2. Stir and serve immediately.

JUICY FACT

This wildly healthy juice increases red blood cell count and lowers blood pressure. It cleanses your blood, organs, and gastrointestinal tract of debris and stimulates metabolism. It also aids in reducing blood pressure by dilating the blood pathways throughout the body.

Potent Juice Elixirs

In This Chapter

- Nutritious and energizing elixirs
- Warming and toning juice combinations
- Potent healing potions

Who didn't love tinkering around in their kitchen as a child making elixirs and potions? (Some of us still do!) Of course, the results probably weren't edible, but we can still have a little fun in the kitchen as adults. The juice elixir blends in this chapter combine the benefits of fresh juices with the therapeutic qualities of more potent ingredients like medicinal herbs, spices, and wheatgrass.

These recipes have been formulated to take your juice fast to the next level. In this chapter, you'll find delicious yet healing elixir blends to warm you from the inside, stimulate detoxification, cleanse your blood, and enhance your immune system. You could actually do an entire juice fast using only these recipes, and you'd find the results absolutely incredible!

Apple Lemon Cinnamon Elixir

This flavorful combo is satisfying, slightly warming, and very energizing. This juice tastes like a fragrant homemade apple pie.

Yield:	Prep time:	Serving size:
about 2 cups	15 minutes	2 cups
Each serving has:		
387 calories	86 g carbohydrates	1 g fat
8 g fiber	2 g protein	8% vitamin A
107% vitamin C	11% calcium	11% magnesium
9% iron	25% potassium	

4 medium Fuji or honeycrisp apples, cored and sliced	1 medium-small lemon, outer rind removed, white pith intact, and sectioned
	2 tsp. ground cinnamon

1. In a low-rpm juicer, alternate pressing Fuji apple slices and lemon sections.

2. Gently stir cinnamon into juice.

3. Serve immediately.

JUICY FACT

Cinnamon has incredible health benefits. Studies have shown it regulates blood sugar, reduces LDL (bad) cholesterol levels, fights against
bacteria and other pathogens, and reduces pain linked to arthritis.

Lemon Ginger Apple Reishi Elixir

A sweet and delicious combination, this anti-aging juice has a zingy yet earthy taste. You'll feel energized and euphoric after just one glass.

Yield:	Prep time:	Serving size:
about 2 cups	15 minutes	2 cups

Each serving has:		
317 calories	85 g carbohydrates	1 g fat
7 g fiber	3 g protein	6% vitamin A
117% vitamin C	6% calcium	10% magnesium
7% iron	21% potassium	

3 medium Fuji apples, cored and sliced	1 (1-in.) piece peeled fresh ginger
1 medium lemon, outer rind removed, white pith intact, and sectioned	20 to 30 drops reishi tincture (nonalcoholic)

1. In a low-rpm juicer, alternate pressing apple slices, lemon sections, and ginger.

2. Gently stir reishi tincture into juice.

3. Serve immediately.

JUICY FACT

Reishi extract is exceptionally high in antioxidants and is known to have incredible anti-aging benefits. It has been shown to lower blood pressure, reduce chronic fatigue, and cure a variety of skin disorders. Reishi also is purported to help fight cancer.

Coconut Wheatgrass Shiitake Elixir

A refreshing vital blend of liquid sunshine, this island favorite tastes mildly pungent and sweet.

Yield:	Prep time:	Serving size:
about 2 cups	15 minutes	2 cups

Each serving has:		
106 calories	20 g carbohydrates	1 g fat
5 g fiber	4 g protein	0% vitamin A
34% vitamin C	12% calcium	30% magnesium
28% iron	34% potassium	

2 cups young coconut water	20 to 30 drops shiitake tincture (nonalcoholic)
¼ cup wheatgrass juice	

1. Pour young coconut water into a jar.

2. Gently stir wheatgrass juice and shiitake tincture into coconut water.

3. Serve immediately.

JUICY FACT

Shiitake extract has been proven to boost the immune system, protect against cancer, and improve the appearance of skin, thanks to such an abundance of antioxidants.

Lemon Ginger Cayenne Goji Stevia Elixir

From the minute this powerful juice hits your throat, you'll know you're about to transcend, with a sweet zipping flavor that's sure to keep you bouncing.

Yield:	Prep time:	Serving size:
about 2 cups	15 minutes	2 cups

Each serving has:		
221 calories	53 g carbohydrates	1 g fat
4 g fiber	4 g protein	172% vitamin A
430% vitamin C	20% calcium	9% magnesium
27% iron	18% potassium	

8 medium lemons, outer rind removed, white pith intact, and sectioned	⅛ tsp. cayenne
	21 drops goji berry extract
1 (1-in.) piece peeled fresh ginger	2 drops liquid stevia extract

1. In a low-rpm juicer, alternate pressing lemon sections and ginger.

2. Gently stir in cayenne, goji berry extract, and liquid stevia extract.

3. Serve immediately.

JUICY FACT

Goji berries are full of amino acids and essential fatty acids. They also contain a remarkable concentration of antioxidants that help combat premature aging, with 10 times more antioxidants than red grapes and 10 to 30 times the anthocyanins of red wine.

Carrot Pear Mint Lucuma Hemp Seed Oil Elixir

This juice is flavorful and grounding. The mint balances the sweetness of maplelike lucuma, while the hemp oil provides a nutty-tasting tincture that will have you coming back for more.

Yield:	Prep time:	Serving size:
about 2 cups	15 minutes	2 cups

Each serving has:		
602 calories	73 g carbohydrates	28 g fat
8 g fiber	4 g protein	817% vitamin A
45% vitamin C	11% calcium	13% magnesium
8% iron	32% potassium	

4 medium-large carrots	2 tsp. powdered lucuma
2 small pears, cored and sliced	2 TB. cold-pressed hemp seed oil
6 fresh mint sprigs	

1. In a low-rpm juicer, alternate pressing carrots, pear slices, and mint.

2. Gently stir in powdered lucuma and hemp seed oil.

3. Serve immediately.

JUICY FACT

Hemp seed oil contains an ideal balance of omega-3 and omega-6 fats for sustainable health. It has a full amino-acid spectrum, provides complete protein, and has a massive trace mineral content—truly one of nature's superfoods.

Apple Holy Basil Tomato Cilantro Elixir

This stress-releasing elixir will leave you with an incredible feeling of emotional well-being. The flavor is similar to a home-cooked Italian tomato soup—very yummy!

Yield:	Prep time:	Serving size:
about 2 cups	15 minutes	2 cups

Each serving has:		
279 calories	74 g carbohydrates	1 g fat
5 g fiber	3 g protein	42% vitamin A
82% vitamin C	5% calcium	12% magnesium
7% iron	30% potassium	

3 medium Granny Smith apples, cored and sliced

1 large tomato, sliced

8 sprigs cilantro

30 drops organic holy basil extract

1. In a low-rpm juicer, alternate pressing Granny Smith apple slices, tomato slices, and cilantro.

2. Gently stir in holy basil extract.

3. Serve immediately.

JUICY FACT

Holy basil (also known as tulsi) extract is effective in helping minimize the effects of stress and promote mental clarity. It also contains lots of antioxidants. As a side benefit, the strengthening qualities associated with the antioxidants help the body's immune system function at full efficiency.

Açai Maca Shilajit Stevia Cacao Elixir

This juice is extremely powerful, combining an array of strong flavors to create an overall sweet and creamy taste with a hint of earthiness.

Yield:	Prep time:	Serving size:
about 2 cups	15 minutes	2 cups

Each serving has:		
277 calories	19 g carbohydrates	14 g fat
5 g fiber	6 g protein	47% vitamin A
63% vitamin C	13% calcium	17% magnesium
10% iron	19% potassium	

1 cup frozen açai berry purée	20 to 30 drops shilajit tincture
1 cup filtered water	15 drops stevia extract
1 tsp. maca powder	1 TB. raw cacao powder

1. In a high-speed blender, combine frozen açai berry purée, water, maca powder, shilajit tincture, stevia extract, and raw cacao powder.

2. Blend on low setting until creamy and smooth.

3. Serve immediately.

TANTALIZING TIP

This concoction isn't a typical juice, but more of a thin fruit purée. We recommend trying it during your cleanse because of its healing bene-fits. It's best to drink this the day before you break your fast because it might trigger your hunger.

Mangosteen Pau D'Arco Pineapple Elixir

Tropical and exotic, this herbal juice blend has a wonderful sweet, tart flavor that blends perfectly with mild pau d'arco.

Yield:	Prep time:	Serving size:
about 2 cups	15 minutes	2 cups

Each serving has:		
574 calories	138 g carbohydrates	3 g fat
11 g fiber	6 g protein	14% vitamin A
689% vitamin C	15% calcium	37% magnesium
19% iron	35% potassium	

½ small pineapple, peeled, cored, and sliced	12 fresh mangosteen fruits or 3 TB. powdered mangosteen fruit
1 medium Fuji apple, cored and sliced	30 drops pau d'arco tincture

1. In a low-rpm juicer, alternate pressing pineapple slices, Fuji apple slices, and mangosteen fruit (if using).

2. Gently stir pau d'arco tincture and mangosteen powder (if using) into juice.

3. Serve immediately.

JUICY FACT

Mangosteen is an incredible energy booster with anti-aging properties. It has been used to treat diarrhea, urinary tract infections, eczema, and dysentery. Pau d'arco is used to treat toxicity and is extremely cleansing. It has been shown to fight bacterial, viral, and parasitic infections.

Noni Ginger Apple Cider Vinegar Cayenne Elixir

This juice is extremely cleansing and has a pungent salty, tart, spicy flavor. It boasts quite a kick and will definitely wake up your taste buds.

Yield:	Prep time:	Serving size:
about 2 cups	15 minutes	2 cups
Each serving has:		
39 calories	9 g carbohydrates	0 g fat
1 g fiber	1 g protein	10% vitamin A
373% vitamin C	224% calcium	55% magnesium
2% iron	237% potassium	

1 medium fresh noni fruit, hand-pulverized in a nut milk bag, juice reserved, and seeds removed, or 2 TB. powdered	1 (2-in.) piece peeled fresh ginger
	1 TB. apple cider vinegar
	Dash cayenne
	1 cup filtered water

1. In a high-speed blender, combine noni juice/purée, ginger, apple cider vinegar, cayenne, and filtered water.

2. Serve immediately.

Variation: Noni has a very pungent flavor. Try adding 1 tablespoon maple syrup if you find the flavor unpleasant.

TANTALIZING TIP

You can buy ripened noni at most Asian supermarkets. To prepare, wash the fruit without bruising the skin while cleaning it. You may use the fruit fresh or transfer it into an airtight sealed container to begin the aging and fermentation process. Leave the container outdoors for at least 6 to 8 weeks to ferment and separate the pulp and juice. This increases the healing benefits of the fruit.

Pear Turmeric Lemon Elixir

This healing tonic is sweet, slightly bitter, and a tad sour. The combination creates a taste sensation that's both delicious and extremely healing.

Yield:	Prep time:	Serving size:
about 2 cups	15 minutes	2 cups

Each serving has:		
427 calories	113 g carbohydrates	2 g fat
12 g fiber	4 g protein	4% vitamin A
104% vitamin C	9% calcium	17% magnesium
24% iron	31% potassium	

4 medium-small pears, cored and sliced	1 (3-in.) piece peeled fresh turmeric
1 medium lemon, outer rind removed, white pith intact, and sectioned	

1. In a low-rpm juicer, alternate pressing pear slices, lemon sections, and turmeric.

2. Serve immediately.

JUICY FACT

Turmeric is a culinary spice that's been proven as a preventive agent for a wide range of diseases, due largely to its anti-inflammatory properties. It can be used to treat cancer and other degenerative diseases.

Orange Strawberry Echinacea Elderberry Elixir

Tart elderberry and the tangy, sweet combination of strawberry and orange are the cold-busting medium for immune-enhancing echinacea.

Yield:	Prep time:	Serving size:
about 2 cups	15 minutes	2 cups

Each serving has:		
232 calories	46 g carbohydrates	2 g fat
6 g fiber	5 g protein	18% vitamin A
422% vitamin C	17% calcium	14% magnesium
6% iron	25% potassium	

3 medium oranges, outer rind removed, white pith intact, and sectioned	20 drops echinacea tincture (nonalcoholic)
	2 TB. prepared elderberry syrup
10 medium strawberries, green leaves intact	

1. In a low-rpm juicer, alternate pressing orange sections and strawberries.

2. Gently stir echinacea tincture and elderberry syrup into juice.

3. Serve immediately.

JUICY FACT

Elderberry is an excellent aid to alleviate detox symptoms during your cleanse. This nutritional powerhouse is also abundant in antioxidants. Echinacea is known to build the immune system and prevent seasonal colds and flus.

Apple Carrot Orange Gingko Ginseng Elixir

This sweet and citrusy yet earthy tonic is extremely health promoting. It'll leave you with boundless energy.

Yield:	Prep time:	Serving size:
about 2 cups	15 minutes	2 cups

Each serving has:		
189 calories	45 g carbohydrates	1 g fat
4 g fiber	3 g protein	618% vitamin A
128% vitamin C	11% calcium	10% magnesium
5% iron	27% potassium	

3 medium carrots

1 medium-large Fuji apple, cored and sliced

1 small orange, outer rind removed, white pith intact, and sectioned

28 drops gingko biloba tincture (nonalcoholic)

28 drops ginseng tincture (nonalcoholic)

1. In a low-rpm juicer, alternate pressing carrots, apple slices, and orange sections.

2. Gently stir gingko biloba tincture and ginseng tincture into juice.

3. Serve immediately.

JUICY FACT

Gingko biloba has been used for centuries to promote mental clarity, alertness, and focus. It has been shown to improve memory, too. Ginseng is used to increase physical and mental endurance, boost energy, normalize body functions, reduce cholesterol, and prevent cancer. Traditionally, ginseng has been used to enhance sexual desire by promoting the production of sex hormones.

Apple Cucumber Burdock Elixir

This mildly sweet, mellow tonic has earthy overtones and is extremely grounding.

Yield:	Prep time:	Serving size:
about 2 cups	15 minutes	2 cups
Each serving has:		
273 calories	66 g carbohydrates	1 g fat
6 g fiber	3 g protein	7% vitamin A
43% vitamin C	7% calcium	15% magnesium
7% iron	24% potassium	

3 medium-small Fuji apples, cored and sliced

½ medium cucumber, sliced

1 (5-in.) piece fresh burdock root, scrubbed clean

1. In a low-rpm juicer, alternate pressing apple slices, cucumber, and burdock root.

2. Serve immediately.

JUICY FACT

Burdock root is loaded with cancer-curing properties. The root also has been used as a remedy for scalp problems, and it purifies the blood, which is essential during your cleanse.

Pear Cucumber Vitamineral Green Elixir

This drink is mildly sweet and savory with an earthy aftertaste.

Yield:	Prep time:	Serving size:
about 2 cups	15 minutes	2 cups

Each serving has:		
348 calories	89 g carbohydrates	1 g fat
8 g fiber	5 g protein	198% vitamin A
74% vitamin C	23% calcium	37% magnesium
43% iron	29% potassium	

4 small pears, cored and sliced	2 TB. Vitamineral Green
½ medium cucumber, sliced	

1. In a low-rpm juicer, alternate pressing pear slices and cucumber slices.

2. Gently stir Vitamineral Green into juice.

3. Serve immediately.

JUICY FACT

Vitamineral Green is a nutritionally dense, therapeutic green superfood powder that supports detoxification and blood sugar balance; tones the liver and kidneys; detoxes the blood, colon, and pancreas; builds bones and muscles; improves immune function, brain function, and circulation; and increases longevity. No wonder it's a superfood!

Juices from the Masters

In This Chapter

- Healing juices
- Specialty juices
- Famous juice blends
- Potent herbal tonic juices

The "secret" juices in this chapter cover a plethora of potent restorative qualities that hold the keys to healing countless health problems. Many of these juices have been favorites of restaurant-goers, and others have been used as the cornerstones for recovering from illness. Some of these juices boast exotic flavors, and others are among the most nourishing and balancing juices you'll ever taste.

We've compiled this collection of revered juices from the leaders in the juicing world to give you a taste of the amazing flavors and healing attributes of well-designed juice combinations. We want you to have the best of the best in your repertoire during your juice fast, so we've searched far and wide to bring you all of the most amazing juice blends on the planet.

Hollywood Celebrity Juice Blend

This brilliantly colored pink juice blend is famous for its syrupy pineapple bite that perfectly complements earthy beets and bright spearmint.

Yield:	Prep time:	Serving size:
about 4 cups	15 minutes	4 cups

Each serving has:		
475 calories	95 g carbohydrates	1 g fat
3 g fiber	5 g protein	23% vitamin A
407% vitamin C	13% calcium	22% magnesium
17% iron	30% potassium	

½ medium-small red beet, sliced

2 large Granny Smith apples, cored and sliced

½ large pineapple, peeled, cored, and sliced

3 medium sprigs spearmint

1. In a low-rpm juicer, alternate pressing red beet slices, Granny Smith apple slices, pineapple slices, and spearmint.

2. Stir and serve immediately.

JUICY FACT

This was the most popular drink served at the renowned Source Restaurant on Sunset Boulevard in the 1970s. The restaurant was one of the first all-organic venues in the world, and many Hollywood celebrities dined there, hence the name of the juice. At the time, though, this drink was named the Hollywood Sunset.

Muscle-Builder Juice Blend

This savory, power-building juice is bursting with flavor. A medley of some of the most nutritious and tasty flavors out there, we recommend you drink it before or after a workout during your juice fast.

Yield:	Prep time:	Serving size:
about 4 cups	15 minutes	4 cups

Each serving has:		
364 calories	45 g carbohydrates	16 g fat
6 g fiber	7 g protein	699% vitamin A
224% vitamin C	20% calcium	25% magnesium
16% iron	62% potassium	

5 medium-small ripe tomatoes, sliced	1 small lime, outer rind removed, white pith intact, and sectioned
3 medium celery stalks	
3 medium carrots	Large handful small blueberries
1 medium lemon, outer rind removed, white pith intact, and sectioned	1 TB. cold-pressed flaxseed oil
	½ cup filtered water

1. In a low-rpm juicer, alternate pressing tomatoes, celery, carrots, lemon sections, lime sections, and blueberries.

2. Gently stir flaxseed oil and filtered water into juice.

3. Serve immediately.

JUICY FACT

This juice was inspired by the documentary *Fat, Sick, and Nearly Dead*, which details Joe Cross's personal mission to regain his health. Joe used the power of juice fasting to lose weight. He even was able to throw away his medications after fasting reversed his chronic ailments.

Blossoming Lotus Juice Aide

The simple ingredients in this fresh green juice create an exotic combination. This sweet, herbal drink is a wonderful departure from mundane juice blends.

Yield:	Prep time:	Serving size:
about 4 cups	15 minutes	4 cups

Each serving has:		
611 calories	120 g carbohydrates	2 g fat
9 g fiber	3 g protein	23% vitamin A
122% vitamin C	11% calcium	18% magnesium
12% iron	38% potassium	

5 large Fuji apples, cored and sliced	1 (2-in.) piece peeled fresh ginger
1 medium lime, outer rind removed, white pith intact, and sectioned	20 medium-large fresh basil leaves
	7 large sprigs cilantro

1. In a low-rpm juicer, alternate pressing Fuji apple slices, lime sections, ginger, basil leaves, and cilantro.

2. Stir and serve immediately.

JUICY FACT

This juice is served in Oregon's Blossoming Lotus restaurant, co-owned by our very own Bo Rinaldi. This is an all-time favorite signature offering in the restaurant and is revered for its Thai-inspired flavors.

Tropical Paradise Juice

This scrumptious juice will transport you to a stress-free tropical paradise. This juice explodes with bright, sunny flavors, leaving you in total bliss.

Yield:	Prep time:	Serving size:
about 4 cups	15 minutes	4 cups

Each serving has:		
523 calories	96 g carbohydrates	2 g fat
8 g fiber	6 g protein	76% vitamin A
974% vitamin C	22% calcium	38% magnesium
16% iron	59% potassium	

1 medium ripe papaya, peeled, seeded, and sliced	1 (1-in.) piece peeled fresh ginger
	1 medium kiwi, peeled
1 small pineapple, peeled, cored, and sliced	½ cup fresh young coconut water

1. In a low-rpm juicer, alternate pressing papaya slices, pineapple slices, ginger, and kiwi.

2. Gently stir coconut water into juice.

3. Serve immediately.

JUICY FACT

This juice was a chance discovery at a roadside juice stand on the beautiful island of Kauai. Although the juice stand is no longer in business, we're happy to share this recipe and keep this best-selling juice alive. It's simply incredible.

Brahman's Best Juice

This tangy and slightly sour ancient elixir has a pungent gingery bite. It's intensely purifying.

Yield:	Prep time:	Serving size:
about 4 cups	15 minutes	4 cups

Each serving has:		
310 calories	52 g carbohydrates	2 g fat
7 g fiber	5 g protein	72% vitamin A
267% vitamin C	17% calcium	24% magnesium
45% iron	34% potassium	

3 small mangoes, peeled and sliced away from pit	1 (2-in.) piece peeled fresh turmeric root
2 medium lemons, outer rind removed, white pith intact, and sectioned	1 (1½-in.) piece peeled fresh ginger
	15 medium-large sprigs mint
	2 cups filtered water

1. In a low-rpm juicer, alternate pressing mango slices, lemon sections, turmeric root, ginger, and mint.

2. Gently stir filtered water into juice.

3. Serve immediately.

JUICY FACT

This ancient recipe originated in India about 5,000 years ago and was used by Rishis and Brahmans as a preparation for worship. It's no wonder, either—this juice is divinely purifying!

Café Gratitude Potion

This juice is nourishing and satisfying, with a spicy, sweet, and slightly savory taste that's earthy and grounding.

Yield:	Prep time:	Serving size:
about 4 cups	15 minutes	4 cups

Each serving has:		
512 calories	103 g carbohydrates	1 g fat
10 g fiber	3 g protein	22% vitamin A
80% vitamin C	11% calcium	18% magnesium
9% iron	42% potassium	

5 medium Fuji apples, cored and sliced	2 large celery stalks
½ small red beet, sliced	1 (1-in.) piece peeled fresh ginger

1. In a low-rpm juicer, alternate pressing Fuji apple slices, red beet slices, celery, and ginger.

2. Stir and serve immediately.

JUICY FACT

Café Gratitude serves delicious, 100 percent organic vegan and raw vegan meals throughout California. They support local famers, sustainable agriculture, and environmentally friendly products. Each café offers an assortment of juices, and this juice, which they call I Am Worthy, is one of the best.

Emerald Lemonade

An incredible alternative to traditional lemonade, this nourishing juice is a delicious blend of sweet, tart, and zesty. You'll love it!

Yield:	Prep time:	Serving size:
about 4 cups	15 minutes	4 cups

Each serving has:		
581 calories	120 g carbohydrates	3 g fat
12 g fiber	8 g protein	635% vitamin A
552% vitamin C	52% calcium	44% magnesium
36% iron	69% potassium	

4 medium Fuji apples, cored and sliced	2 medium cucumbers, sliced
1 medium lemon, outer rind removed, white pith intact, and sectioned	4 medium kale leaves
	2 TB. organic raw agave nectar

1. In a low-rpm juicer, alternate pressing Fuji apple slices, lemon sections, cucumber slices, and kale leaves.

2. Gently stir organic raw agave nectar into juice.

3. Serve immediately.

JUICY FACT

Real Food Daily was founded in 1993 by vegan chef Ann Gentry. The two locations in Southern California offer a 100 percent vegan menu, exclusively using food grown with organic farming methods. They also offer fresh organic juices any time of the day. This emerald lemonade is one of our favorites.

Druid's Detox Juice

This juice should be a staple during your juice fast. The earthy and subtly bitter flavors balance perfectly with a touch of heat and mild sweetness.

Yield:	Prep time:	Serving size:
about 4 cups	15 minutes	4 cups

Each serving has:		
639 calories	121 g carbohydrates	2 g fat
13 g fiber	6 g protein	8% vitamin A
125% vitamin C	30% calcium	44% magnesium
23% iron	53% potassium	

2 large burdock roots, scrubbed clean	1 (1-in.) piece peeled fresh ginger
4 medium Granny Smith apples, cored and chopped	2 TB. organic raw agave nectar
1 medium lemon, outer rind removed, white pith intact, and sectioned	Dash cayenne

1. In a low-rpm juicer, alternate pressing burdock roots, Granny Smith apple slices, lemon sections, and ginger.

2. Gently stir organic raw agave nectar and cayenne into juice.

3. Serve immediately.

JUICY FACT

Leaf Organics founder Rod Rotondi serves Druid's Detox as part of his raw food and vegan menu at his Los Angeles restaurant. A leader in the raw-food and green movement, Rod also distributes a Leaf Organics packaged food line in health stores across the country.

Patricia Bragg's Best Juice

This is a delicious, ideal pick-me-up. The juice has a zesty, tart kick balanced by a sweet, lingering aftertaste.

Yield:	Prep time:	Serving size:
about 4 cups	15 minutes	4 cups

Each serving has:		
418 calories	107 g carbohydrates	0 g fat
0 g fiber	0 g protein	0% vitamin A
0% vitamin C	13% calcium	7% magnesium
11% iron	256% potassium	

½ cup Bragg's organic apple cider vinegar	32 drops organic herbal stevia
½ cup grade B 100 percent organic maple syrup	3 cups filtered water

1. In a high-speed blender, combine Bragg's organic apple cider vinegar, organic maple syrup, organic herbal stevia, and filtered water.

2. Blend on low for a few seconds until thoroughly combined.

3. Serve immediately.

JUICY FACT

Paul Bragg and his daughter, Patricia, have been health pioneers for decades. When fast food captured the attention of most Americans, Paul campaigned for a diet and lifestyle that focused on natural live foods and a healthy regimen for a vital and long life. These ideas, based around natural and organic foods, are gaining praise and acceptance world wide. This was one of Paul's favorite drinks.

Jay Kordich's Must-Have Juice

This juice is a delicious summer tonic. The flavor is sweet and yet just a bit tart, perfect to drink on a beautiful sunny day.

Yield:	Prep time:	Serving size:
about 4 cups	15 minutes	4 cups

Each serving has:		
547 calories	117 g carbohydrates	3 g fat
9 g fiber	9 g protein	117% vitamin A
545% vitamin C	13% calcium	33% magnesium
20% iron	58% potassium	

3 medium ripe peaches, pitted and sliced	1 medium pineapple, peeled, cored, and sliced
6 ripe apricots, pitted and sliced	1 (½-in.) piece peeled fresh ginger

1. In a low-rpm juicer, alternate pressing peach slices, apricot slices, pineapple slices, and ginger.

2. Stir and serve immediately.

JUICY FACT

Jay Kordich has recommended this juice for years, praising its ability to tone the skin, plus its anti-inflammatory properties and its excellent blood-building qualities. It also protects the heart against all sorts of maladies.

açai The small, deep purple, phytonutrient-rich berry of the *Euterpe oleracea* palm tree, a native to the Amazon region in South America. It's well known for its high antioxidant content and is used in smoothies and juices and as a blend served with granola.

acid-forming food Food such as meat, eggs, milk, cheese, grains, and beans that lowers the body's pH, creating an acidic environment. Acid-forming foods can increase the risk of osteoporosis, asthma, and kidney problems.

adaptogen A plant food or herb used to rejuvenate and balance the body. It's also said to reduce the effects of stress, anxiety, and trauma on the body.

alkaline-forming food Plant food such as fruits and vegetables that raise the body's pH toward its ideal level of 7.4 pH.

alkalinity Refers to a pH that's greater than 7, which is neutral. In this book, alkalinity refers to the pH of human blood in particular. The proper pH for human blood is between 7.2 and 7.8, which is slightly alkaline.

aloe vera A succulent plant, actually in the lily family, whose clear, inner leaf is commonly used as a folk remedy for treating external wounds and burns and a variety of digestive and degenerative diseases.

antioxidant A protective phytochemical that blocks the harmful effects of oxidation on cells. Numerous plant substances, including vitamins and phenols, have antioxidant properties.

Ayurveda   A traditional form of medicine originated in India and believed to have been used for more than 5,000 years. Its premise is to restore balance based on one's body type and uses different mineral and plant medicines to achieve this. It may also make recommendations for certain yoga postures or changes to one's lifestyle.

B vitamins   A family of eight vitamins including thiamin, riboflavin, niacin, pantothenic acid, pyridoxine, biotin, B_{12}, and folic acid we require for metabolism, healing, and a healthy nervous system.

cayenne   A fiery spice made from hot chile peppers, especially the cayenne chile, a slender, red, and very hot pepper.

cellular respiration   The process by which cells utilize energy by breaking the bonds in ATP (the simple sugar used for energy production by the body) molecules and then removing the waste products from these chemical changes.

chelator   A substance that binds a chemical or other element and suppresses its chemical activity.

chia seed   An ancient seed originating in South America that has a unique, energy-giving composition of 31 grams fat, 38 grams fiber, and 16 grams protein per 100 grams.

chlorella   A type of single-celled algae cultivated for its beneficial health properties. It's a rich source of protein, vitamins, minerals, and essential fatty acids.

cider vinegar   A vinegar produced from apple cider, popular in North America.

cilantro   A member of the parsley family used in Mexican dishes (especially salsa) and some Asian dishes. Use in moderation because the flavor can overwhelm. The seed of the cilantro plant is the spice coriander.

cinnamon   A rich, aromatic spice commonly used in baking or desserts. Cinnamon can also be used for delicious and interesting entrées.

conventional   Refers to food products and/or methods of growth and production that use pesticides, herbicides, antibiotics, and other artificial chemicals.

detoxification   The natural or accelerated process by which the body removes toxic substances in an effort to reach homeostasis (a state of normal equilibrium).

dill   A pungent herb.

Echinacea purpurea* and *augustifolia   The most commonly used species of this immune-stimulating plant.

electrolyte   Essential minerals including calcium, magnesium, sodium, and potassium the body requires to regulate cellular communication and water transfer and to maintain muscle function.

enteric nervous system   A peripheral aspect of the nervous system that governs digestion and sends messages to the brain that effect mood and well-being.

fiber   The nondigestible substance in the cell walls of plants that acts as a cleansing agent in the body, promoting good digestion and encouraging detoxification.

free radical   A toxic atom containing unpaired electrons that attacks and damages human cells. They promote heart disease and inflammatory illnesses such as arthritis and Alzheimer's.

garlic   A member of the onion family, a pungent and flavorful vegetable used in many savory dishes. A garlic bulb contains multiple cloves. Each clove, when chopped, provides about 1 teaspoon garlic.

genetically modified   Designation for plants whose genes have been artificially altered to induce certain characteristics, such as disease or drought resistance. The long-term effects of genetic modification on human health are unknown, so these foods are best avoided.

ginger   A flavorful root available fresh or dried and ground that adds a pungent, sweet, and spicy quality to a dish.

ginseng   An adaptogenic herb generally prepared from the dried and powdered root of the Panax ginseng plant.

green smoothie   Smoothies that include leafy green vegetables mixed with fruit as part of their ingredients.

high-speed blender   A blender with higher voltage and Hz than a traditional blender. It has the capacity to powder nuts, crush ice, and reduce nearly any vegetable, fruit, or green to a creamy, silky texture.

homeostasis   The physiological processes that help to maintain a state of equilibrium in a living organism.

inflammatory disease   An illness such as arthritis, asthma, blindness, and dementia caused by inflammation of body tissues.

macronutrient   The main energy-providing components (calories) of human nutrition: carbohydrates, protein, and fat.

mangosteen   The small, white-fleshed fruit of the *Garcinia mangostana* tree native to Indonesia. The fruit is housed inside a hard, thick purple rind and contains edible seeds. While the fruit portion of the plant is used for various folk remedies, it's the deep purple rind that gives mangosteen products their purple color and phytonutrient value.

maqui berry   A small purple-black berry with an impressive antioxidant content—one of the highest levels known. The polyphenols in these berries carry a variety of antioxidant and cancer-fighting benefits.

micronutrient   The component part of macronutrients that provide noncaloric nutrients—that is, vitamins, minerals, enzymes, and phytonutrients.

nettle   The stinging nettle (*Urtica dioica*). Nettles have a diuretic effect helpful for the kidneys and also aid arthritis and anemia. They grow throughout North America and should be handled with care to avoid being stung.

organic   Foods produced without the use of artificially manufactured pesticides, herbicides, and fungicides.

oxidation   The browning of fruit flesh that happens over time with exposure to air. Minimize oxidation by rubbing the cut surfaces with lemon juice.

oxidative damage   The damage caused to cells and DNA by free radicals as a result of oxygen exposure.

parsley A fresh-tasting green, leafy herb, often used as a garnish.

pH Refers to the chemical balance of a solution. Water is neutral at 7 pH, while basic solutions have a pH higher than 7 and acidic solutions have a pH lower than 7. The ideal pH for human blood is between 7.2 and 7.8, which is slightly basic.

phytochemical A chemical compound found in any plant that may have healing or toxic effects on the body depending on the nature of the chemical. Phytochemicals give color, smell, and flavor to plant foods and can indicate whether or not a plant is edible.

phytonutrient A chemical compound found in fruits and vegetables that plants produce to protect themselves and are also beneficial to human health. They include carotenoids, flavonoids, sulphides, isoflavones, capsaicin, and lycopene.

pinch An unscientific measurement for the amount of an ingredient—typically, a dry, granular substance such as an herb or seasoning—you can hold between your finger and thumb.

psyllium husks The outer covering of the seed of the *Plantago ovate* plant. They expand and become gelatinous when soaked in water.

reishi mushroom (*Ganoderma lucidum*) A mushroom with almost supernatural powers of health and healing. It contains terpenes and polysaccharides that make it useful in treating cancer and autoimmune diseases. It's bitter tasting, and the powdered mushroom may be easily mixed into other foods to mask its flavor.

super-greens powder A high-quality blend of different powdered grasses like wheatgrass or barley grass that may also contain various herbs like nettle or horsetail. Some super-greens powders also contain probiotics and enzymes.

tonic As referred to in this book, a tonic is an herbal substance that promotes general health or invigorates particular organs in the body.

turmeric A spicy, pungent yellow root used in many dishes, especially Indian cuisine, for color and flavor. Turmeric has tremendous anti-inflammatory properties and is the source of the yellow color in many prepared mustards.

vegan Refers to a plant-based lifestyle free of animal and animal-derived products and foods such as meat, fish, eggs, dairy, honey, gelatin, and rennet.

wheatgrass juice The pressed juice of the wheat berry sprout, *Triticum aestivum*. Wheatgrass is reputed to be an effective treatment for diabetes, hypertension, and cancer. It chelates heavy metals and has superb nutritional qualities that correct many deficiencies.

Resources

Now that you're empowered with the knowledge that will enable you to juice fast with great success, you can check out these further resources to get the tools and support you need to get started or deepen your commitment to the juice-fasting lifestyle.

Juicing Books

Airola, Paavo. *Juice Fasting: The Age-Old Way to a New You!* Sherwood, OR: Health Plus Publishers, 1971.

Brown, Ellen. *The Complete Idiot's Guide to Juicing.* Indianapolis, IN: Alpha Books, 2007.

Burroughs, Stanley. *The Master Cleanser.* Reno, NV: Burroughs Books, 1976.

Ehret, Arnold. *Rational Fasting for Physical, Mental and Spiritual Rejuvenation, Fifteenth Edition.* Dobbs Ferry, NY: Ehret Literature Publishing Co., Inc., 1994.

Gerson, Charlotte, with Beata Bishop. *Healing the Gerson Way: Defeating Cancer and Other Chronic Diseases, Second Edition.* Carmel, CA: Gerson Health Media, 2010.

Kirschner, Dr. H. E. *Life Food Juice: For Vim, Vigor, and Vitality, Thirtieth Edition.* Monrovia, CA: H. E. Kirschner Publications, 1975.

Kordich, Jay. *The Juiceman's Power of Juicing.* New York, NY: Time Warner Books, 1993.

Lus, John B. *Raw Juice Therapy.* New York, NY: Benedict Lust Publications, 1956.

Meyerowitz, Steve. *Juice Fasting and Detoxification: Use the Healing Power of Fresh Juice to Feel Young and Look Great, Sixth Edition*. Great Barrington, MA: Sproutman Publications, 1999.

———. *Wheatgrass: Nature's Finest Medicine: The Complete Guide to Using Grasses to Revitalize Your Health, Sixth Edition*. Great Barrington, MA: Sproutman Publications, 1999.

Morse, Robert. *The Detox Miracle Sourcebook*. Prescott, AZ: Hohm Press, 2004.

Shelton, Herbert. *Fasting Can Save Your Life, Sixth Edition*. Tampa, FL: American Natural Hygiene Society, Inc., 1996.

Walker, Dr. Norman. *Fresh Vegetable and Fruit Juices: What's Missing in Your Body? Revised Edition*. Prescott, AZ: Norwalk Press, 1981.

Cookbooks for Your Transition Menu

Abrams, Maribeth. *The 4 Ingredient Vegan*. Summertown, TN: Book Publishing Company, 2010.

Boutenko, Victoria. *Green for Life*. Ashland, OR: Raw Family Publishing, 2005.

Gentry, Ann. *The Real Food Daily Cookbook*. Berkeley, CA: Ten Speed Press, 2005.

Reinfeld, Mark, Bo Rinaldi, and Jennifer Murray. *The Complete Idiot's Guide to Eating Raw*. Indianapolis, IN: Alpha Books, 2008.

———. *Vegan Fusion World Cuisine: Extraordinary Recipes and Timeless Wisdom from the Celebrated Blossoming Lotus Restaurants*. New York, NY: Beaufort Books, 2007.

Rinaldi, Bo. *The Complete Idiot's Guide to Green Smoothies*. Indianapolis, IN: Alpha Books, 2012.

———. *The Complete Idiot's Guide to Low-Fat Vegan Cooking*. Indianapolis, IN: Alpha Books, 2012.

Soria, Cherie, Brenda Davis, and Vesanto Melina. *The Raw Revolution Diet.* Summertown, TN: Book Publishing Company, 2008.

Waltermyer, Christine. *The Natural Vegan Kitchen.* Summertown, TN: Book Publishing Company, 2011.

Books That Support Healthy Lifestyle Change

Campbell, Colin T., and Thomas M. Campbell II. *The China Study: The Most Comprehensive Study of Nutrition Ever Conducted and the Startling Implications for Diet, Weight Loss, and Long-Term Health.* Dallas, TX: Benbella Books, 2006.

Cousens, Gabriel. MD. *Conscious Eating.* Berkeley, CA: North Atlantic Books, 2000.

———. *There Is a Cure for Diabetes.* Berkeley, CA: North Atlantic Books, 2008.

———. *Rainbow Green Live Food Cuisine.* Berkeley, CA: North Atlantic Books, 2003.

———. *Spiritual Nutrition: Six Foundations for Spiritual Life and the Awakening of Kundalini.* Berkeley, CA: North Atlantic Books, 2005.

Esselstyn, Caldwell. *Prevent and Reverse Heart Disease.* New York, NY: Avery, 2007.

Graham, Dr. Douglas N. *The 80/10/10 Diet.* Key Largo, FL: FoodnSport Press, 2006.

Klein, David. *Self Healing Colitis and Crohn's.* Sebastopol, CA: Colitis and Crohn's Health Recovery Center, 2006.

Kulvinskas, Victoras. *Survival into the 21st Century: Planetary Healers Manual.* Woodstock Valley, CT: 21st Century Publications, 1981.

Marcus, Erik. *Vegan: The New Ethics of Eating.* Ithaca, NY: McBooks Press, 2001.

Ornish, Dean. *Dr. Ornish's Program for Reversing Heart Disease: The Only System Scientifically Proven to Reverse Heart Disease Without Drugs or Surgery.* New York, NY: Ivy Books, 1995.

Robbins, John. *Diet for a New America.* Tiburon, CA: HJ Kramer, 1987.

Wigmore, Ann. *The Hippocrates Diet and Health Program.* New York, NY: Avery, 1983.

Juicing Videos

Fat, Sick, and Nearly Dead: The Joe Cross Movie
fatsickandnearlydead.com

May I Be Frank
mayibefrankmovie.com

Juice-Fasting Community Support

Juice Guru
juiceguru.com
(This is Steve Prussack's juicing website featuring videos and inspirations to stay motivated and juicing.)

Juice-Fast Experts
juicefastexperts.com
(This is our online juicing support coaching and buddy-up program.)

Juice Hotline
juicehotline.com

Juicer Sources

Juice Fast Supplies
juicefastsupplies.com

Herbs and Other Helpful Ingredients

Botanical Preservation Corps.
botanicalpreservationcorps.com/store

Golden Lotus Botanicals
goldenlotusherbs.com

HealthForce Edge Cleanse and Longevity Boxes
healthforcebox.com

Medical Professionals Who Support Juice Fasting

Dr. Cousens' Tree of Life Rejuvenation Center
treeoflife.nu

Dr. Schulze
herbdoc.com

Radical Healing
radicalhealing.com

Healing Centers and Retreats

Gerson Institute
gerson.org

Hippocrates Health Institute
hippocratesinst.com

An Oasis of Healing
anoasisofhealing.com

Optimum Health Institute
optimumhealth.org

Rancho La Puerta
rancholapuerta.com

Tree of Life
gabrielcousens.com

Websites to Support Your Health Journey

Colitis and Crohn's Health Recovery Center
colitis-crohns.com

Cooking Healthy Lessons
cookinghealthylessons.com

Go Dairy Free
godairyfree.org

Green Smoothie Challenge
greensmoothiechallenge.com

Happy Cow
happycow.net

Jay Kordich's School of Juicing
schoolofjuicing.com

Juice Fast for Health
juicefastforhealth.com

Rawpalooza
rawpalooza.com

Vegan Fusion Cuisine
veganfusion.com

Vegan Meetup Groups
vegan.meetup.com

Veganpalooza
veganpalooza.com

Vitamix
vitamix.com

We Care Spa
wecarespa.com

World Peace Diet Mastery Program
worldpeacemastery.com

Stories of Transformation

In this appendix, we've collecting some moving and inspiring stories of healing and transformation from a few generous individuals who volunteered their stories hoping to inspire others. As enthusiasts of the juice-fasting lifestyle and the authors of this book, you'll find both of our personal healing stories as well.

These experiences give you a window to the awesome effects of juice fasting. We hope these testimonials to the powerful effects of juice fasting inspire you to find what miraculous changes you can make in your life.

Steve: Whole-Life Transformation

By the time I graduated college 20 years ago, I was a mess. College life was fun, living in a fraternity house and taking advantage of all the indulgence around me. I had no idea what "health" even meant, and laughed at the vegetarians in the cafeteria. It was beyond my imagination how anyone could eat just plant foods. Are these people crazy? Why don't they eat real food? The junk-food diet I was on for the majority of my life was starting to take its toll. I was overweight, suffered from migraine headaches, severe seasonal allergies, low depression, and an overall negative disposition. Help was on the way.

A couple years out of college, I knew I had to make a change. I was out of breath climbing a few stairs in a building! I hated looking at my body and would usually hide behind clothing and towels. I didn't want to look at my body naked. It revealed too much. Yet one night I took a hard look at myself. I didn't like what I saw. I began researching health, in between smoking a pack of cigarettes a day and drinking a six-pack of beer. I began to exercise. It wasn't long before I discovered the power of juicing. I decided to try a juice fast.

My first one was 3 days, and I thought I was going to die! It seemed like I was juicing for a year! I couldn't wait to eat food again. This short-term fast didn't do much to improve my health. I dropped a couple pounds but then I immediately resumed my poor diet choices.

As my diet began to evolve, I started to eliminate all the foods that were clearly leading to my ill health. I cut out the milk and dairy. I began to eat only organic free-range meats. Still, I wasn't feeling great. I was in my early 20s, yet was tired all the time. I was depressed. Life just wasn't going great.

Finally, I embarked on a few intermittent juice fasts. Mainly, I followed the lemonade diet (Master Cleanse) and saw noticeable results. My weight began to drop. I became more intuitive. When I would finish a fast, I had cravings for *healthy* food! I became vegetarian, then eventually vegan, and finally raw vegan.

Although I was vegan/raw vegan, I still had high cholesterol. I couldn't understand it. I thought I was eating well. I was exercising, had quit smoking, and was doing all the things I thought I should to improve my health. The change came when I started juicing again and went through a detox that changed my life.

I was in my late 30s, working as an occupational therapist with autistic children. I decided to start juicing for a few days. I wasn't sure how long I was going to fast; I just knew I wanted to drop the extra fat around my belly and hopefully get my cholesterol down. My body went into a major healing crisis and started pouring years of accumulated junk out of my body. The most profound thing happened. I had given up smoking more than 15 years before this cleanse and exercised just about every day. Yet one morning I noticed the tips of my fingers were starting to peel. I looked closer, and saw black soot coming out of the tips of six of my fingers! I inspected the soot, smelled it, and found it was actually nicotine coming out of my body! It was stored in my fat cells and finally was being released thanks to a raw food diet and juice fast!

It didn't end there. My body went into a total elimination mode. I was in the bathroom every hour and couldn't have a normal movement. I began to panic, wondering if I had taken this too far. Why couldn't I have a solid bowel movement? I checked into the hospital where they ran a battery of tests. To my amazement, the results indicated I was in phenomenal health and shape. Better yet, I found that my cholesterol had finally dropped, and for the first time, it was actually low!

My life had changed. I became happy, less moody, more energetic ... it was easy to get out of bed in the morning. I was able to develop loving relationships without fear. My mind became sharper. My focus became better.

These changes convinced me that everything I read about juicing and raw foods was true. This really was the best way to live, and my body was clearly letting me know.

Today, I fast quarterly (four times a year) and in addition include a "one-time-a-week" juice/water fast to keep me on track. My body continues to let go of the years of abuse. During every cleanse, I release more and more mucus and toxic waste. I would have had disease by now, had I not found this lifestyle. I would have been like the many others, living on medications and eating unconsciously.

The changes keep coming. On my last cleanse of 23 days, my body balanced to the point where I no longer get migraine headaches! My body is trim, and I have the same level of energy as when I was a teenager. My energy might be even better now. I improve my diet more and more after every cleanse. My intuition tells me what I need to eat, and I am slowly letting go of emotional attachments to food. It's not always easy. We have been conditioned to eat for comfort since we were babies. Comfort foods do more than fill the stomach; they're tied to the limbic system, and our early memories are triggered with the foods we eat. It takes work to start new and clear away those attachments. We begin to find comfort in a glass of organic juice, or a meal of lettuce or fruit.

I can't put into words the gratitude I have for finding the juice-fasting lifestyle. I am happy to share my passion with you through this book and others to come. I'm glad you decided to try juice fasting. You can expect the same changes—physically, emotionally, mentally, and spiritually.

Bo: Healed at Age 12

I have been a vegan since 1960. At the age of 12, my mother and father were beside themselves, as I had seemingly incurable asthma and allergies. We went to every clinic and doctor they could find, yet no one was able to help me. Then in 1960, my mother took me to a Seventh Day Adventist doctor who gave her the book *Back to Eden*. I read the book from cover to cover, and in 2 weeks, I was a budding herbalist and vegan cook, not even knowing what those terms meant! In a matter of 2 weeks, I reversed *all* the symptoms of my asthma and allergies and have enjoyed perfect health since. I eliminated all the wheat, dairy, eggs, and meat and am forever grateful to that doctor, my beautiful mother, and yes, all who have helped me on my path.

Growing up in Southern California, I had access to a great education, wonderful resources, and a beautiful environment. I could feel the beginning of the health-food movement in the early 1960s even then. I was a precocious kid, and I learned that the term *vegetarian* was not in our language until 1839, and that before that we were called *Pythagoreans*. I believe, as did Pythagoras, that the "man-to-plant" connection is the ultimate way to human perfection. The man who brought us the theory of 7, the golden mean, pi, and many other ideas related to numbers, also brought us the wisdom that the color of food describes its workings in our bodies! Sound familiar? Modern-day science is just catching up to Pythagoras with discoveries about superfoods, phenols, and the healing nature of color in our food sources. Maybe this will inspire you to invite your 12-year-old into the kitchen to learn the ancient art of preparing a plant-based feast.

I am now in my 60s, never use any medicine, am healthier than ever, and am blessed with a beautiful wife and family. I have been blessed to author many books on this subject of healthy diet through a vegan lifestyle, and one of the most important topics in my journey was learning and applying the benefits of juice fasting.

Along my path of health and healing, I met many incredible people. I was fortunate to be an integral part of the organic natural food movement of the California 1960s. I was able to meet and work with such incredible people as Dr. Bronner, Dr. Bernard Jensen, Dr. Paul Bragg, and Stanley Burroughs. My main mentor was Dr. Pietro Rotundi, who was the doctor who assisted John Lennon in the *Lost Years* when John lived in Laurel Canyon. Suffice it to say, what I learned and experienced in those days fuels me even to this day.

My first recollection of juice fasting was when I was 9 years old and my grandmother read the book *The Grape Cure* by Johannes Brandt. That one moment, when I began to think about just simply living on juices for curative and restorative purposes, was the beginning of a deep realization for me. Indeed my first long fast of 40 days was an all-fresh grape juice fast that defined the mystical aspects of this approach. I learned so much about juice fasting from Victor Irons, who introduced the concepts of what the Native Americans used for their ritualistic cleansings, through the use of Bentonite, a product you can still buy at your local health-food store.

As I tried many fasting techniques, from the watermelon fast to the grapefruit diet, I must say they all had equal effects on me—a deep and profound calming of my energy, quickening of my mind, and fortification of my spirit. As such, I have been able to offer my expertise, both personal and professional, to many thousands of folks who also seek these benefits. As simple as this may seem, it can be quite difficult without a system, a path, a support group or a great work, such as what we offer in this book.

I love to fast annually, generally for a "spring cleaning." I also sometimes fast on Sundays, utilizing that day for rest and restoration, which is quite natural given the busy life we seem to lead during every moment of our lives. However, when I think about fasting, I remember what Stanley Burroughs taught me in 1974 on the island of Oahu. I was working with Stanley on the healing aspects of color, and how the color of food affects our organs and health. We exposed freshly squeezed lemonade to colored lights in a special room he had made. We then tested the "charged" lemonade on ourselves and our friends for its possible curative effects. Stanley was adamant that this alone could help our entire humanity and that we needed to bring the color back into our lives.

It was from these teachings that he shared with me his thoughts regarding the Master Cleanse, probably the number-one fasting technique ever shared. He said that the yellow of the lemon would activate our solar plexus, the red pepper our blood and digestion, and the gold of the maple syrup our higher centers. Now, I don't believe anyone can really prove this scientifically. However, if you go on a Master Cleanse for 10 days, I know you'll experience what Stanley called "the clearing." Whenever I go on a Master Cleanse, I not only lose weight and feel purer than ever, I also feel clearer of mind than ever. I think Stanley was on to something, and I know for a fact, the colors of food do indeed teach us what their properties might be, as mentioned earlier, in regard to their active phenol content.

While many fast for a specific purpose, I notice one common thread regarding fasting. I fast to calm myself, to give my body a rest, and to restore my being, and I must say it always works. It is for this reason alone that I am eternally grateful to be able to share the knowledge I have gained regarding all the various recipes, techniques, and programs with my co-author Steve Prussack with anyone interested in rejuvenating themselves using this safe and wonderful approach to health.

Dr. Thomas Lodi: An MD's View on Juicing

Health can only be obtained by living within the biological laws that govern our bodies. If one desires to build anything, three basic things are required: the blueprint (plan), the materials, and someone to do the work. This is as true for our bodies as it is for inanimate objects.

We already have the blueprint, our DNA, which requires raw materials and energy. There are trillions of cells that make up our bodies. Millions of cells are dying and being replaced every minute and all the others are engaged in countless numbers of reactions that keep us functioning. But these processes require a constant flood of materials (nutrients), including all the macronutrients and micronutrients as well as oxygen, water, and sunlight.

When the appropriate materials are not available, substitutes are utilized or incorporated. For example, the cell walls (the "skin" of your cells) need fats. If the appropriate omega fatty acids are not available, oxidized (rancid) fats or "stiff" (trans-fatty acids) are incorporated into the cell walls. The result is a poor, malfunctioning membrane. Your body will utilize whatever it has available to it in order to maintain operational functioning of the whole.

Consequently, our cells are regenerated with defective materials and are largely unable to function. As these defective cells continue to be produced, organs deteriorate and what is known as "chronic disease" ensues. The solution to "disease" then becomes obvious when viewed from this perspective. Assist the body in expelling all of the inappropriate materials and ensure that appropriate materials are made available. Quite simple, actually.

The quickest way this can be achieved is to literally flood the body with nutrients by taking more raw materials than could be eaten in a day and turn them into juice so that they can be consumed. One quart of fresh vegetable juice provides more nutrition than the average American gets in six months to one year. So if one drinks several quarts per day, the body has abundant materials to perform its work. The necessity of assisting in the removal ("detox") of unusable materials also becomes obvious to one with a clear understanding of how biological entities function. The activities that one can incorporate to assist in this regard include, but are not limited to, colon hydrotherapy, lymphatic drainage techniques (including exercise), yoga, and proper and adequate sleep (renewal of organs of elimination).

A fellow from the west coast of the United States came to our center with stage-4 lung cancer, which carries an extremely dismal prognosis. He drank four to five quarts per day of fresh, green vegetable juice, and within five weeks a PET scan was unable to detect any active cancer. The same has occurred with stage-4 pancreatic cancer, as well as every other cancer, albeit in differing amounts of time. Of course, this is not all that they were doing, but those who don't happily and gratefully do a green juice feast do not get these results. The same rate and depth of healing occurs with all other chronic conditions such as diabetes, high blood pressure, arthritis, digestive malfunctions, and others.

Because "fasting" means to take into the body nothing but water, we refer to juicing (without eating) as "juice feasting," because it results in mega amounts of nutritional substances being made available for renewal and regeneration.

Karen Sinclair: Healing Deadly Lesions

I am currently on day 56 of a 92-day juice *feasting* journey to whole life health. I prepared myself by transitioning to a low-fat, raw, organic vegan diet. My health greatly improved from just doing the transition. My body fat percentage was too high and this is why my naturopathic physician and I agreed that doing a juice fast would be the next step.

I've gotten off caffeine, which was a miracle in itself. I knew going into this adventure that eliminating caffeine would be part of the program. Glad I did. My liver loves me for it. I no longer suffer from fatty liver disease. I no longer suffer from glucose resistance/muscle fatigue/seizures. My face is 95 percent cleared up from pre-cancer lesions. I have a 30-year history of skin cancer. This is a miracle!

My sleep is fantastic. My energy level is stable and high. My thinking is clear and focused. My nails are growing for the first time in my life. Clarity of my life's purpose has never been as clear. I am more patient, more loving and understanding. My desire to be involved with others has skyrocketed! I was a loner and still do enjoy my solitude, however my involvement with others has quadrupled.

I have had several bouts of strong detox symptoms. Some of these were surprising. Others weren't. Enemas are necessary and help the body eliminate the stored toxins. I have changed as a person in such radical ways. I am not the same woman who started this journey. Who I will be when I reach day 92? I'm certain I will be glorious!

Mark Gstoh: Reversing Diabetes

In September 2011, I was drastically overweight and as a type-2 diabetic could not control my blood sugar. I saw the film *Forks Over Knives* and thought I'd give veganism a try. Within a month, I'd lost quite a bit of weight, but more importantly I had gone from taking four pills a day for my blood sugar to only one a day and my blood sugar was completely under control! Since that time I learned about juicing through *Raw Vegan Radio*. It's a great way to get all of the nutrients I need and in a terrifically tasty way as well.

I've made juicing a regular part of my diet because it's good for me and I've been surprised at how great the juices taste. Although some friends and family think my lifestyle has become a bit too radical, it's really hard to argue with the results. I continue to lose weight and I feel a lot better, not only because I weigh less, but because I am eating better!

I'm very motivated to continue my new lifestyle, not only for me but also for my family and friends. I want to become more of an advocate for juicing and veganism because I know it makes an impact on one's health and on our world. This "kind diet" is good for our planet in so many ways! As a professor of theology, I'm developing a course on the theology of food so that I can introduce my students to the various religious practices related to vegetarianism and veganism. I can't wait to teach the class so that I can have students sample fresh vegetable juice and learn about the various benefits of meatless diets and diets free from animal products.

Raw Vegan Radio is an excellent resource for my new lifestyle! The information and resources available have helped me to avoid common mistakes and have encouraged me to explore new ways to enjoy different foods.

Index

Numbers

A

B

S

Y-Z